OUTSMART YOUR DIABETES:

A Step-by-Step Guide to Reversing Type 2 Diabetes

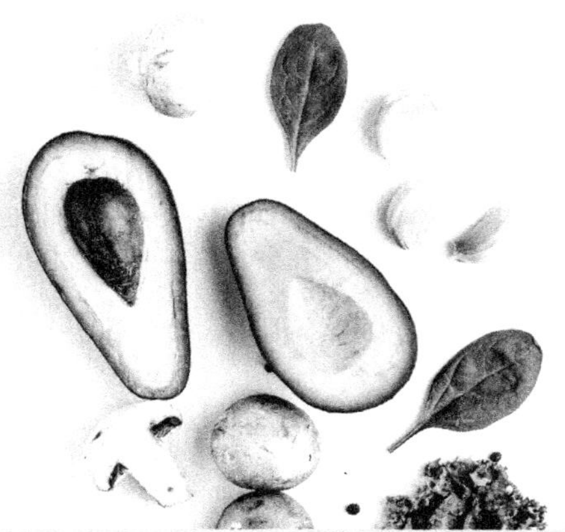

ANGELA MANDERFELD RD

Diabetes Nutrition Expert

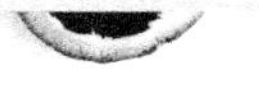
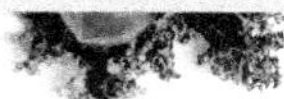

Grateful Clients

Angela's program helped me change to a healthy lifestyle. I was able to stop several of my diabetes medications and lost weight. I'm working on achieving my goal, which is to maintain a well-controlled diabetes with healthy diet and exercise without medications. The challenges are easy to understand and very informative. I will continue because it makes me feel great and energetic. I have tried several diet programs and failed. But this works!

—AK Be

I was diagnosed 2 years ago with type 2 diabetes. I have lost 3 immediate family members due to health issues related to diabetes. Since being diagnosed I have participated in Weight Watchers (several times) as well as Eat Less Move More. Angela provided far better tools that I could walk away with and apply daily.

—Outsmart Your Diabetes Program Participant

I would highly recommend Angela's programs to anyone that has an interest in Diabetes!

—Outsmart Your Diabetes Program Participant

In December 2016, I was diagnosed with Type 2 Diabetes and my Doctor prescribed medicine for the diabetes. Angela helped me to change my lifestyle and my diet. She taught me to make healthy food choices and also motivated me to get moving and exercise. Through her help, I lost weight and my A1c came down.

My A1c came down so much, that within 6 months my Doctor took me off of diabetes medicine. I feel like what I have learned I can continue. Angela has taught me that my "medicine of choice" is healthy eating and exercise!

—Beth P.

I've learned so much about nutrition, about my body and mind, and how all those things come together to provide me with a healthier perspective. I wholeheartedly believe that I have made positive changes for the long term.

—Kim B.

Angela taught me a lot about how to diversify my meals and how to fuel my body. This is not about making you feel bad about food choices but to bring awareness. I feel so much better after making small but impactful changes, such as adding more veggies and snacking less. You do have to put in the work and time and I feel I achieved my goals because of that. I can happily continue putting into practice the tools that I learned. If you're thinking of doing one of Angela's programs, you won't regret it!

—W.M.

Dedication

To my mom, you inspire me, I love you.

To Sam, you can do anything you put your mind to, "love you so much."

Introduction

Writing this book was a daunting endeavor for me. I had to face the fears of judgment, criticism and failure. I know that many people with diabetes share those same fears. How often have you shared your diabetes diagnosis and been given unsolicited advice or criticism of food choices, because "someone with diabetes shouldn't eat that?" This book will give you the tools, the peace of mind, and the power you deserve to manage both your food choices and your diabetes. I am honored that you are holding this book in your hands and I want you to know that I care about you and your health.

This is not a "cure" or quick fix for diabetes. It is, however, designed to break down the overwhelming task of reversing diabetes - but with a twist. You will end up with an individualized approach to reverse your course toward diabetes. I will take you one step at a time through the process. If you have type 2 diabetes and want to take charge of your blood sugar and your health, this book is for you. If you are sick of following diet after diet and not getting the results you want, this book is for you. Diabetes may someday become your reality, but the extent to which it impacts your life can be controlled.There is much to cover as we move ahead. I recommend reading a little at a time and writing down your action plans in a dedicated notebook. If you start to get overwhelmed – slow down! Focus on what resonated with you and take time to get comfortable with it. You may be excited to forge ahead, but you also want to allow what you've learned to become familiar and natural. This will help sustain your progress. Remember – slow and steady wins the race. Food is medicine. Ultimately, the goal is to acquire all the benefits that food can provide to achieve the healthiest lifestyle possible.

Join me on this journey to optimal health with diabetes. I am your guide, so strap in, hold on and enjoy this quest, as we shift this life as you know it, and throw diabetes in reverse.

With gratitude,

Angela

Table of Contents

CHAPTER 1

The What, Who, I, and Why of Reversing Diabetes

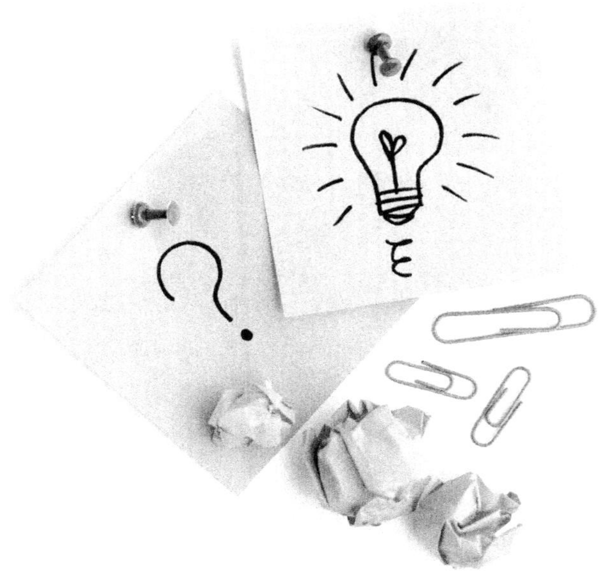

I recall a time about 23 years ago sitting in my grandparents' basement at a clunky old computer helping my grandpa create an Excel spreadsheet of his morning and bedtime blood sugars to bring to his medical appointments. He liked to take this report to show how well he was doing with his blood sugar control, always hoping to get a "thumbs up" from his doctor. Today we have apps, continuous glucose monitors (CGM) and smart phones for monitoring blood sugar trends. Before all this, the little blood-stained notebook with dates and handwritten blood sugars was how it was done. That little notebook represented whether my grandpa had been "good" or "bad" — or at least that's how he saw it.

My grandpa loved food. Why wouldn't he? My grandma was an amazing cook. Angel food cake with strawberries was his favorite. He believed it was "good for his diabetes" (probably because it was low-fat).

If he was still with us, grandpa would be in his early 90's. I wish he hadn't spent so much of his life with diabetes, feeling guilty about his diet. If only he had the opportunity to eat meals that were healthy, delicious, and above all...kept his blood sugars in target range.

While the technology has improved, I really wish many other things had changed in the years since my grandpa was diagnosed with diabetes. For example: people checking their blood sugar for themselves rather than their doctors, no longer passing judgement on themselves because of what they ate in a day, and I wish everyone knew that low-fat and fat-free eating is not the way to manage diabetes.

Fast forward 18 years. I am sitting with my mom in the kitchen as she looks at a CGM she will wear for the next week. She sees a number register in the 170 mg/dl range and I see panic on her face. She didn't even have a diagnosis of diabetes – yet.

My parents left their own home for 3 years to move in with and care for my other grandpa with Alzheimer's. During this time, my mom was under so much stress, she would often break down in tears. She was tired, had little energy and decided to go back to work (after retirement) thinking it would help alleviate her problems. Her weight was increasing slightly, her stress level was high, and she and my dad would often eat out just to take a break. Given her genetic predisposition and stressful lifestyle, at this point, a diagnosis of diabetes was inevitable. She would listen to my recommendations and sometimes make changes, but was not yet able to commit.

As we sat in my kitchen that day and looked at her 170 mg/dl reading on the CGM, she began to quiz me about what was making it go that high and how she could get it down. I gave her a few ideas, one of which was to start moving after meals. The next thing I knew, she was walking circles through my house with my 3-year-old in tow in an effort to make her blood sugar come down. She lost 5 pounds that week and when she returned home, she continued walking, losing weight, and driving down her numbers.

Her mindset changed, motivation grew, and her transformation accelerated exponentially. She would not go to bed at night until her smart watch hit 10,000 steps. She was eating differently and joined an exercise studio. As much as I would love to take credit for all the amazing things she did, her transformation was a personal, conscious decision to live a quality lifestyle, to be around to enjoy her grandkids, and to not have high blood sugar. Once she decided to kick diabetes, my dad jumped right on board with her. Together they created a support system which enhanced her progress and desire to succeed. My dad walks with her daily and also eats a healthier diet.

At the time of her diagnosis, my mom's A1c test result was 6.7%. The doctor started her on medication. At her three-month checkup, her A1c had dropped to 5.7%. She and her doctor agreed to a trial off the medication. This challenge increased her motivation even more. By the following checkup, while continuing her 10,000+ steps each day, attending 7 classes a week (yoga, muscle conditioning, Zumba), and practicing mindful eating, she had lost a total of 20 pounds.

A note about the A1c test: it's a blood test that estimates

average blood sugar by telling us what percentage of red blood cells have sugar attached. Normal is <5.7%; prediabetes is 5.7%–6.4%; 6.5% and up is a diagnosis of diabetes.

My mom will often mention her fear of what would happen if she stopped doing all that she's doing. I reassure her that it's different this time. Recently, she told me how she feels a little selfish; everything is all about her now. I reassure her again... it should be all about her. Between you and me, the way I know that she is really serious and that this change is permanent is this: when we would visit her, she'd skip her classes or not go walking because she wanted to spend that time with her grandson. Now, when we visit, she gets up early and walks daily, does pool exercises, and still spends time playing with her grandson. She incorporates exercise into her daily routine now to feel confident she will have time with her grandkids in the future.

Fighting against diabetes can be hard. It can produce feelings of denial, anger, and self-doubt. Yet once the decision to manage it is made, it can induce feelings of hope, confidence, and control. Diabetes may be a part of your life, but you have the opportunity to achieve harmony with it.

I get really frustrated with books that keep you in suspense over the course of innumerable chapters before revealing their secrets. So I am going to give you six actions you can take right from the start. These are not rules for life, but rather are steps designed to raise your awareness about certain behaviors that could be driving up your blood sugar. By understanding and practicing these behaviors at the outset, I strongly believe you will see changes while you continue to read this book. Please remember, what works for your neighbor or your best friend is not necessarily what is going to work for you. You need to take the time to individualize this and really think about what is important to you.

That said, I ask you to trust this process and yourself to give your body and soul what they need without relying on rules and willpower. There's simply no reason to wait until the book's end to begin... so let's get started.

The SECRET

Remember, these are not rules you have to live by forever. Rather, these are steps to raise awareness of certain habits that may be impacting your blood sugar. Think of them as tools to achieve the results you deserve.

S

SNACKING

This can be a dangerous habit and you don't have to do it simply because you have diabetes. Snacking is NOT your friend – at least not right now. It's important to try to avoid eating between meals so you can establish "true" hunger. Hunger is that feeling when your stomach is telling you that it's time for food. More on this later.

Eat only at meal times and then notice if you start to experience feelings of hunger before your next meal. If you do and it's TRUE hunger – that physical feeling in your gut that you need food – it's acceptable to have a small snack. A good snack could be a cup of vegetables with hummus or avocado, or a handful of berries and a few nuts. Keep it small and simple and remember – the goal is to be hungry again by your next meal.

E

END WITH CARBOHYDRATES

A small study showed that when people ate the carbs last, their post-meal blood sugar levels were about half as high as when they ate carbs first. This equated to blood sugars typically 40% lower than when the subjects ate all food groups together. The carbohydrate-last meal was also associated with lower insulin secretion and higher levels of glucagon-like peptide-1 (GLP-1), a gut hormone that helps regulate blood sugar and satiety. Save carbohydrate foods like rice, potatoes, bread, pasta and other starches for last. It helps prevent overeating and slows the rise in blood sugar. To achieve a better benefit, be a carbohydrate snob and only choose carbohydrates that have a decent amount of fiber like fruits, vegetables, whole grains, and beans. The other carbs are not worthy of you (at least not on a regular basis).

We will talk about individualization and specifics later. This is just a general recommendation to get started on the right foot. Try saving the carbs for last! Make sure you check your blood sugar before your meal, and again two hours after your meal, to see if this is working for you.

C

CHEW FOOD SLOWLY

Slowly chew your vegetables and meat first. Really taking time to chew improves your digestion. I once heard someone advise chewing each bite for a minute, but that seems like overkill. Instead chew your food slightly longer than normal. Wait until you've fully swallowed before loading your fork again. This little change will help reduce the sense of urgency for that next bite. Since we are talking about slowing down, this is a good time to suggest taking a few deep, cleansing breaths to calm the body before you eat. Just take a moment to relax.

R

REPLENISH FLUIDS

Choosing drinks that are not sweet will keep your energy up and your blood sugar down. Flavored, unsweetened tea (my mother-in-law introduced me to Tazo Glazed Lemon Loaf tea that tastes like dessert) and "spa" water are great ways to stay hydrated and boost levels of antioxidants and vitamins.

Examples of spa water are those with mint and cucumber/tarragon, or cucumber/lemon and rosemary. Choose whatever herbs and fruits sound appealing to you. Carry a 20 oz. or larger water bottle. Aim to drink 60-90 oz. of water a day (where you live, your activity level, and your body weight will impact how much fluid you may need in a day).

E

ENERGY BURN

Most people like to relax after dinner. One of the worst choices you can make is to be sedentary after a meal. Moving around for 10 minutes after each meal could help lower your blood sugar. Don't think of this as formal exercise. Rather than sitting, reading or watching TV shortly after a meal, plan some activities that require movement such as household chores like washing dishes, laundry, vacuuming or walking the dog. Make a list of activities that require movement for 10 minutes after you eat. Once dinner is over, set the timer and go for it.

Just knowing you will be active after eating may help direct your attention to that satisfied feeling and avoid becoming overly full.

Important note: Just to be clear, movement after a meal is not to "burn calories" because you just ate. The purpose of moving after a meal is to aid digestion and help process any carbohydrates you may have consumed. Movement helps get sugar out of the blood and into your cells, therefore lowering your blood sugar.

T

TIMING

Avoid eating after 7 or 8pm, then don't eat again for 13 hours. Wait, what? I know what you're thinking — people with diabetes are "supposed" to snack or avoid prolonged periods without eating, right? Also, didn't a bunch of smart people debunk the idea of not eating after 7pm?

The latest studies show that people who wait 13 hours from dinner to breakfast have lower risk of heart disease and insulin resistance. So, if you don't eat after 8pm and hold out for breakfast until 9am, it does a body good!

Adjust the time frame to fit your schedule. If you are using insulin or taking any medication that could cause a low blood sugar reaction (such as a sulfonylurea like glimepiride, glipizide, or glyburide), you should talk to your provider or dietitian first to make a plan for extra blood sugar monitoring. Plan to do at least 1 or 2 middle-of-the-night checks, and be sure to immediately treat any hypoglycemia (low blood sugar) with some carbohydrates such as 4 oz. of fruit juice or a few crackers. Be sure to let your provider know about any low blood sugars so they can adjust your meds. There is no need to feed your medicine. It's better to take less medicine than to eat more food unnecessarily. We will dig a little deeper into the benefits of fasting later on, but this is a simple and great place to get started.

Bottomline:

This is not about starving yourself. It's about giving your body a rest from food and digestion so it can focus on building up your immune system and repairing any breakdown from the day. If you experience true hunger after 8pm and you want to respond with a snack, go for it. In general, not eating at least 3 hours before bed and fasting overnight is good for your system.

Managing diabetes doesn't have to be difficult and, with some creativity, it could even be fun. Consider connecting with a positive support person or accountability partner. Sharing your plan with a partner and then following up with them is a great way to stay motivated. If you find a partner to work with, they don't have to follow the same plan as you, and they don't even need to have diabetes. They simply need a desire to feel better, have more energy and share some accountability.

Many of the recommended actions for managing diabetes are also great for preventing type 2 diabetes. So, even if you have loved ones living with you who don't have diabetes, all will reap the benefits. Pick the easiest of the six actions listed and start today.

Finally, as you work on the SECRET, don't forget to laugh, love and be mindful. Laughing can help lower your blood sugar and help you feel better in general. Additionally, inherent love of yourself and others is motivation to take good care of yourself and that can also lower blood sugar as well. Last, but not least, is mindfulness. When you focus your attention on the present and forget about what happened earlier or what's happening next week, when you give yourself an opportunity to enjoy and experience the here and now, you can do wonders for lowering your blood sugar.

Write down three ways you can incorporate more love, laughter and mindfulness into your daily life and then do it!

Let's take a little time to really understand what is going on in the body with diabetes. When you have an understanding of the inner workings, it helps you understand why you are making the changes. Having a strong reason to do something increases the likelihood that you will do it. Some people will do things because their doctor tells them to, but others need to know why!

What is type 2 diabetes?

Diabetes is when your body cannot process sugar. There are a number of reasons why this may happen. When you eat food, particularly foods that are carbohydrates, your body breaks them down into sugar. Sugar leaves the blood, travels through the fluid between your cells, eventually arrives at a cell, and wants to be let in. Your body makes a hormone called insulin. Insulin acts as a key to open the cell and let the sugar in. On occasion though, the cell will get rid of some of the locks, making it harder for insulin to insert the key and let the sugar in. This is called insulin resistance; the body's cells are being resistant to the insulin it makes. This can cause blood sugar to rise above normal levels.

What puts people at risk of developing type 2 diabetes?

- Having prediabetes
- Being overweight
- Being 45 years or older

- Having a parent, brother, or sister with type 2 diabetes
- Being physically active less than 3 times a week
- Having had gestational diabetes (diabetes during pregnancy) or given birth to a baby who weighed more than 9 pounds
- Being African American, Hispanic/Latino American, American Indian, or Alaska Native (some Pacific Islanders and Asian Americans are also at higher risk)
- Having non-alcoholic fatty liver disease

The secret weapon against stubborn, insulin resistant cells is exercise. Exercise forces the cells to open and allow the sugar to enter. That is why moving around after a meal is so important, even if the movement isn't considered "formal exercise."

Putting large amounts of carbohydrate foods into your system all at once is a lot to process and can overwork the pancreas, causing higher blood sugar. When the sugar stays in the blood and can't get into the cells, the body will start to feel tired and lethargic. The fuel (sugar) is in the body, but it has to get into the cells for us to be able to use it as energy.

Another problem is when people have had high blood sugar for extended periods of time. The pancreas has to work really hard to produce enough insulin to get the sugar into the stubborn cells. When the cells are stubborn, the pancreas actually has to make MORE insulin. So, as I'm sure you can imagine, when the pancreas has to work too hard for too long, it starts to underproduce and gets worn out. The beta cells in the pancreas start to disappear and it loses the ability to keep up the intense "production schedule." Decreasing the amount of carbohydrates eaten at one time, choosing high fiber carbohydrates that do not need as much insulin, and moving the body regularly are all ways to help the pancreas out and reverse diabetes. Sounds simple, right? Well, there's still more to it and we'll cover the nitty gritty in the upcoming chapters.

Who is affected by diabetes?

One in three people has prediabetes and at least 8 out of 10 of those people don't know they have it. There is also research showing that diabetes starts developing as early as 20 years before a person receives their diagnosis. By the time they are diagnosed, their cells have lost at least half of their ability to make an important hormone called insulin, which aids in getting the sugar out of the blood and into the cells where it needs to be.

There was a large study called the Diabetes Prevention Program (DPP) trial which showed that an intensive lifestyle change could reduce the rate of type 2 diabetes by 58% over 3 years. That said, if you are in the prediabetes stage, you have a pretty solid chance of completely reversing it, and that's a big deal.

Another thing you should know is that there is a medication called metformin that is sometimes prescribed for diabetes, but it doesn't work as well as when you change the food you eat and increase the amount you move. More points for the food and movement option!

Here's more hope to consider. Losing only 7% of your body weight can also halt the progression of type 2 diabetes. So let's break that down. A female who is 5'6" and weighs 205 pounds can see significant reduction in diabetes risk by losing ~14 pounds. For a male who is 6' tall and weighs 240 pounds, ~17 pounds of weight loss can slow or stop the progression.

The bottom line is this: small changes make a big difference. The real secret is to take your focus off watching the scale and putting it on the little changes that you can be consistent about.

If you have diabetes, you might not feel any different, much less even know you have it. Many people will have some signs, such as decreased energy, often feeling run down and tired, urinating more (especially in the middle of the night), craving sugar, and feeling drowsy after meals. Many people accept these signs as part of what happens as you age, even though these effects are not considered normal.

So how do I know if I have it?

Below is a chart I created so you can see the different tests that are done to determine your diabetes status. The most common tests to detect diabetes are: hemoglobin A1c, fasting glucose (blood sugar), 2-hour glucose tolerance test, and random glucose. There are other tests such as fasting insulin, but they just provide information and not necessarily a diagnosis.

Always get a copy of your lab work – it's the only way you can really be in charge. The head of a company would never say, "I don't need the financial reports. If you say they're good, they must be good." That would put the fate of the company in the hands of someone else. The same applies to you and your diabetes. Pay attention to your numbers so you can be proactive and not worry about surprises. Sticking your head in the sand and saying "my doctor said I just need to watch my sugar, but I don't have diabetes" is a fast track to getting diabetes. This is your body. You are the "head of the company" trying to keep things on track, so you need all the information possible to stay on top of this. You are the boss. You have hired your healthcare team to provide you with information and support to keep your best interests in mind, but ultimately you are the decision maker because you are the one living with diabetes.

TYPE OF TEST (DONE AT LAB)	NODIABETES	PRE-DIABETES	DIABETES
Hemoglobin A1c (a.k.a. A1c)	less than 5.7%	5.7-6.4%	6.5% or higher
Fasting blood sugar (no food/drink except water for 8 hours)	less than 100 mg/dl	100-125 mg/dl	126 mg/dl or higher
2 Hour Glucose Tolerance Test	less than 140 mg/dl	140-199 mg/dl	200 mg/dl or higher
Random Glucose Test - used when someone has symptoms	n/a	n/a	200 mg/dl or higher

If you get lab work done after fasting and your glucose level on the comprehensive metabolic panel is 100–125 mg/dl, you are in the pre-diabetes range. Don't take comfort if your number comes back at 96 mg/dl. That number is too close to 100 mg/dl to ignore — so the sooner you get on top of it the better.

Two or more of these numbers need to be elevated to make the diagnosis and they can be on the same day or different days. An exception to this rule is if you are exhibiting signs and symptoms of high blood sugar and you have an elevated reading. This could confirm a diagnosis of diabetes.

This chart gives you a better idea of what the A1c really means, by converting it to an estimated average glucose.

A1C%	EAG (ESTIMATED AVERAGE GLUCOSE)
5	97mg/dl (76-120)
6	126mg/dl (100-152)
7	154 mg/dl (123-185)
8	183 mg/dl (147-217)
9	212 mg/dl (170-249)
10	240 mg/dl (193-282)
11	269 mg/dl (217-314)
12	298 mg/dl (240-347)

Your "why" and vision for your health. What happens if you don't reverse diabetes?

Have you ever been told to do something and you think ***"that's crazy... no way!"*** But then you learn why it's important and you start to open up to the idea? I can honestly tell you right off the bat that I'm a "why" person. Each and every task in this book will come with a solid "why" and a solid reason for doing it. Here's the kicker. The general "why" is not going to be good enough unless you have a strong personal "why" for wanting to take steps to avoid diabetes and its complications. That seems obvious, right? No one truly wants diabetes and the complications that can accompany it, so that should be a good enough "why." Agreed?

Of course, that's it right there. A solid "why" is not getting complications from diabetes. Except that it's really not. If simply knowing that you could get complications from high blood sugar was enough to really motivate people, then diabetes would not really be a problem and no one would be struggling. No one actually wants complications, or diabetes for that matter.

Think about it this way: what happens in your life if you don't reverse diabetes? What is it costing you if you don't make a change now? The answer to this question is your "why."

Here's an example:

Why do you want to reverse diabetes? I don't like taking medications.

Why don't you like taking medications? I forget them and I don't like swallowing pills.

Why do you forget to take your medication? I don't like how it makes me feel and it costs so much. If I don't take it every day, I can stretch it out a little further.

Why do you want to stretch it out a little further? Because I don't like having diabetes, I don't want to spend my hard-earned money on medication, and I'm mad that I even have diabetes in the first place.

PAUSE. Let's take a moment and reflect before moving any further in this conversation. The answer to "Why do you want to reverse diabetes?" went from "I don't like taking medications" to "I don't want to spend my hard-earned money on meds and I'm mad that I even have it in the first place". One of those answers is more compelling and motivating than the other. We can even take this a bit further. Let's continue.

Why don't you want to spend your money on medications for managing this disease, even though you are mad you have it? You want to manage it, right? Of course, I want to manage it. I worked hard all my life to have money to travel and I want to see my grandkids. I want to do what I want, when I want, and I don't want to be worrying about taking medications and having to choose between travel or meds. My prescription costs are $700 a month! Plus, now I have to eat like a bird and I can't enjoy my food anymore.

When someone asks why long enough, certain deep-seated feelings surface and you get to the heart of the matter. This person is angry, frustrated, and a little resentful. They want to change, but are a bit scared. Scared they are going to be forced to give up their favorite foods, but also scared they won't spend their retirement the way they dreamed. Emotions are strong motivators for change.

In this situation, some people will just say "forget it" and pretend they don't have diabetes until they can't pretend anymore. Others will say enough is enough and use their "why" to drive them away from diabetes and toward the life they've always dreamed of, but now a life with diabetes. Notice this person did not include answers reflecting worries about a heart attack or how their vision could be affected. Their "why" had nothing to do with complications. Most people don't "want" complications, yet many may be concerned about them. Since we aren't always able to feel them, potential complications just might not be a primary focus. What people can feel is how diabetes affects their wallet or the ability to travel. This is a daily reality. There are other feelings that we have to take into account as well.

Anger is a wildcard when it comes to diabetes. It can send people down a path of denial and spite, or it can light a fire and propel them fiercely in the opposite direction. If you are experiencing anger, denial, guilt, or frustration about having or getting diabetes, you are not alone. For years you probably dreamed of a life full of health and happiness, and diabetes was not in your plans. So when diabetes entered the picture a new reality set in.

So today, grab diabetes and say, "Hey - now that you're here, I'm going to distance myself from you and build a life of peace and harmony between us."

Creating peace and harmony with diabetes can be done with some simple steps. Please remember that just because something is simple, that does not necessarily mean it will be

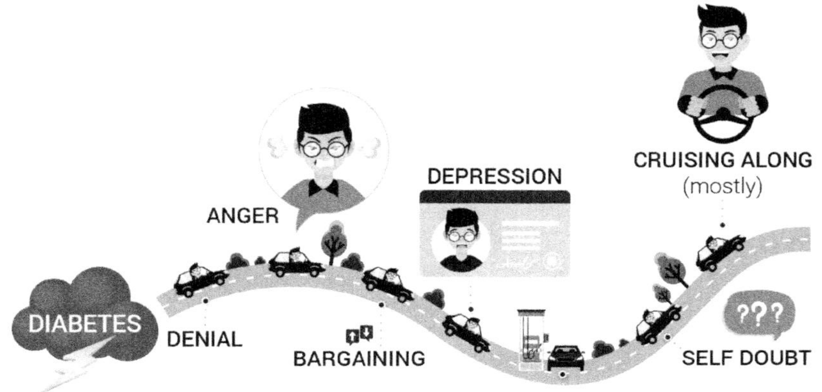

easy. Asking yourself, "Why do I want to do this?" is key. If the reason behind making changes is not strong enough, you may make it one week or maybe even a month and then willpower will be exhausted, leaving a feeling of frustration. If, however, you take some time and drill down to your "why" and make it a strong and powerful statement, it will propel you through the rough times and get you to the end result.

Bottomline:

I don't know the exact number of times you need to ask yourself "Why?" to get to what really drives you, but my guess is that it's at least 5 and might be as high as 25! What's important is that you just start asking.

I've got my "why" so what's next?

Now it's time to decide. You've got your "why," but now you have to actually make the decision to move forward and not look back. Once you've made the decision to move forward, you have a really good reason to do something. Committing and taking action is the next step. Here you will need to think of possible obstacles that will throw you off track. Commit to your health. It's admirable to put everyone else's needs above yours, but it's time to be committed and move yourself to the top of your priority list. It's time and you deserve this.

You owe it to yourself to engage. I'm going to ask a lot of you as we move through this process together. If I ask you to write something down or do something, please don't pretend you are just auditing this book. Get a notebook and start writing. Write down key ideas or suggestions that you want to try before you stop reading. Write at least one small action step that you will start working on immediately. Let go of the excuses of why you can't. Be coachable and just go for it. I'm right here with you.

Understand that you can and will be successful — simply because you decided to. There is no reason why others can do this and you can't. Starting now, prioritize your health by choosing the best for yourself and you WILL be successful.

Put your phone on silent and get rid of distractions. This is time for you and only you. I know it is hard to slow down and focus on yourself, but this knowledge is critical. We are starting on a journey through the what's and why's of diabetes so strap in and stay focused.

You will not be getting a list of rules on what not to do and what not to eat. You will be taking into account your preferences, daily life experiences, likes and dislikes, and from this you will create your individualized plan.

Some of you will choose to start each day with a sweet treat, while others will completely eliminate sugar. Some of you will eat meat and some of you won't. There is no one right answer for everyone. Much of it depends on where you live, what you have access to, and other health conditions. For me to think that I have one solution that will fix everyone would be very presumptuous. However, I will present some general structure

Throughout life, and even during this process, you are going to be tempted to jump on the next "diet" bandwagon. Have you ever been on a roadtrip with a GPS guiding you when suddenly you think you know a shortcut? And before you know it, you're lost and wishing you had paid attention to your GPS? Well, that can happen to any of us at any time. Having a good plan in place, and doing your research ahead of time can prevent getting sidetracked.

and ideas for you to think about. You will then begin your journey to determine what the best approach is for outsmarting your diabetes.

There is a strong pull toward dieting because of what it promises, and because of our desire for instant gratification. "I want results NOW!" We often don't think about long-term effects because we are conditioned to be short-sighted when it comes to our health and, in particular, with regard to body weight. Trust this process because slow and steady wins the race. If you rush through, take on too much, and don't take time to see what works and what doesn't, your results will be short-lived. Stay on course.

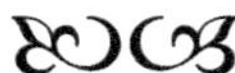

I'd like you to meet Laurie. She came to me because she was really struggling with her weight. She had always been fit and healthy and took pride in that. She was accomplished in her professional life and her grown boys were in college. Laurie loved exercising; she was a great skier, liked biking, and enjoyed taking classes at her local gym.

She had recently separated from her husband and was under a lot of stress. At a recent doctor's visit, Laurie was told she was getting very close to prediabetes. Her recent fasting glucose level was 99 mg/dl and 100 mg/dl marks pre-diabetes.

Laurie had gotten into a habit of eating a really healthful dinner, but then snacking until she went to bed. In the evening she would feel sad and lonely and she began using food to help fill the void.

Perhaps you can identify with Laurie in some way. When she came to me, she was sick of the extra weight and wanted to lose it fast. Quickly I was seeing red flags. She wanted to try intermittent fasting. She had previously experimented with it. She had also adopted bits and pieces of the keto diet, but she stressed her love of starchy carbohydrates (which are contraindicated with keto). She said she was "always hungry," although we could make a strong case that this was not the root cause of the problem.

Hunger is a physical sensation and Laurie soon discovered that after eating a high-quality, balanced dinner, her continued eating was not out of hunger. As Laurie imposed more restrictions on herself, she became more frustrated with her lack of results. Her problem was not the fasting, exercising or choosing healthy food. Rather her problem was eating when she was not hungry in an attempt to remedy her loneliness, stress and sadness. Eating food is the solution when you're actually hungry, but eating is not your friend when you are dealing with emotional issues.

When it comes to weight loss and getting control of our health, we are accustomed to having rules and restrictions related to food. We want someone to tell us what and how to eat. In Laurie's situation, I could have given her perfect meal plans, advised her on portion control, and made sure she had a perfectly balanced diet. None of that, however, would help someone cope with the emotional stress of a personal situation compounded by the stress of having prediabetes. I can't give you a diet to fix the fact that you eat when angry or when stressed, but throughout the book we can look at some effective ways to address those feelings.

We will work on establishing your new normal, not a diet. I will challenge you to uncover what is important and what is not so you can acknowledge habits and why you do what you do. I want you to discover new foods and habits that bring joy to your life. We need to be flexible because life is never going to be "normal." We have all said at one point or another "after this month, things will slow down and get back to normal," or "on Monday, I'll start again." Chances are "normal" may not ever happen. It's important to establish healthy habits now so you can adjust to life's bumps in the road.

Benjamin Hardy, PhD is an organizational psychologist. He has written many blogs and New York Times bestsellers. His work can help many who are struggling to make lifestyle changes. I first learned about the "future self" concept from him and it makes so much sense, especially in diabetes management. Think, taste, feel, and believe that you can be all of the things that you desire. Part of accomplishing that is a vision of your future self. Right now, you might have a less than positive view of yourself. Maybe you tell yourself things like ***"I'm not an exerciser"*** or ***"I'm not a morning person."*** Everyone has some personal belief statements, whether they are general beliefs about who you are as a person or whether they are related to diabetes and health.

What if you could change some of those beliefs? Are there some statements that you would prefer to make about yourself, or some actions that you wish described you? Make a list right now. Grab your journal and write down statements about your desires for your future self. It could be things like: "***I practice yoga daily;***" "***I enjoy being outdoors;***" "***I meditate regularly;***" "***I love cooking.***" You get the idea. Perhaps you hate vegetables but wish you could love them. Write that down. You can make these things happen!

Now write down the priorities in your life such as: family, work, personal growth, health, hobbies, friends, spirituality, money, volunteering, recreation, sports, fitness, home. Pick 3–5 and write them in order of importance. If health or self-care did not make the top 5, you may find it challenging to manage diabetes. I'm not telling you what your priorities should be, but acknowledging your priorities will help you gain a better understanding of the choices you make and how successful you are.

So, let's create a vision of your future self. Make a general statement of your future self and then let's start creating what life looks like for you.

Tell me what life is like for your future self.

What do you do each day? What are your behaviors/routines? How does this make you feel? Be specific.

Write out a perfect (realistic) day. What time do you wake up? How do you feel when you get out of bed? How do you start your day and why? What kind of food do you eat? Where do you enjoy your meals and with whom? What kind of movement do you engage in to enhance your day?

Think hard about your life right now. What do you want more (or less) of in your day? What are the most important things in your life? Do your activities and day-to-day routines exemplify your priorities? If you could change some things, what would they be? Is your job causing you enormous stress because you're working 60 hours a week with no time left for yourself or family? Is this really the way you want to live? Maybe it is. I can't answer that for you. What I can say is that you can achieve change if you have a realistic and attainable vision of what you want out of life. Once you know what you want, you can begin to take steps to get you there. Yes, we are still talking about reversing diabetes, but it's not just about doing what you're told. It's about having a strong desire and vision in order to take the necessary steps.

Let's go deep here for a minute. You have one life to live. Diabetes is now a part of your life. Do you want to live this one life to the fullest or are you going to let life knock you around and deprive you of being the best you can be? This is important. Think of ways you can live your life to the fullest with what you can control. Go back to your "why," look at your priorities, and start making decisions about your life that align with them.

Believe it or not, all of this matters when it comes to diabetes. It matters because as you read this, you either thought — "***YES! I am going to change some things because I want to enjoy this life***." Or you thought "***She's crazy! This is the hand I was dealt and I'm stuck with it.***"

Regardless of your response, you owe it to yourself to keep moving forward, keep trying, keep persevering.

Studies have shown that 95% of what we do today is based on our subconscious, stemming from routines we have developed over the years. Today is the day to stop being passive. Stop doing what you have always done because that's the way you have always done it. Challenge yourself to see and do things differently — take action. This is how you change your health and your life. Obviously, some of the things that occur in your daily life are not ideal or you wouldn't be here with me looking for change. Choose to be proactive and get ahead, rather than sitting back to see what life will throw at you next.

Day by day we live on repeat — not necessarily "Groundhog's Day" kind of repeat — but pretty darn close. What is one thing you could do today to really spice things up in your life and make your day wildly different, fun and productive? Maybe you jump out of bed 30 minutes earlier than usual, run into the bathroom, look at yourself in the mirror, tell yourself how amazing and strong you are, then do 20 minutes of exercise. You're not leaving your house so you don't even need exercise clothes. Just start marching in place, dancing, do some sun salutations — anything that moves your body. For most of us, that would really spice up our mornings and set a whole different pace for the day.

Five ways to take action today:

1. Get up 10 minutes earlier and write down one thing you are grateful for in your life. Then write 3 things you will do for yourself today to intentionally reverse diabetes. For example: eat 1 cup of broccoli at lunch; take a 10 minute walk after dinner; take 3 deep inhales and exhales before I eat.

2. Before you go to sleep at night, plug your phone in to charge in another room. Don't keep it within arms' reach of your bed. You will likely go to bed earlier and sleep better instead of scrolling on your phone. And you will have a better start to your morning because you won't be lying in bed looking at your phone when you are supposed to be getting up.

3. If you normally stop for breakfast on the way to work, plan to make something at home instead, then drive a different route to work. If you work from home, plan to eat breakfast at the kitchen table with no distractions instead of at your desk while checking your email.

4. Take a pause. Pause before you grab candy from the candy jar you walk past every day. Pause before pulling in the drive-thru for coffee. Pause before you hit the snooze button. Pause before you take a second helping at a meal. Pause and do something because you are deciding to, not because it's what you always do.

5. Start and/or end your day with a win. In the morning, make your bed or check your blood sugar; take 5 minutes and do some dinner prep. Before bed, spend 10 minutes tidying up one area in your house; get your clothes or food ready for the next day; think about what you want to accomplish tomorrow. Do something that makes you feel productive and demonstrates that you are making decisions and taking actions that align with your priorities.

I know we have not ***really*** addressed food or activity yet, but the mindset is the groundwork that must be laid, in order for everything else to work. Once we do talk about food and movement, you'll be ready to jump into action.

CHAPTER 2

Is It Really Possible to Reverse Type 2 Diabetes?

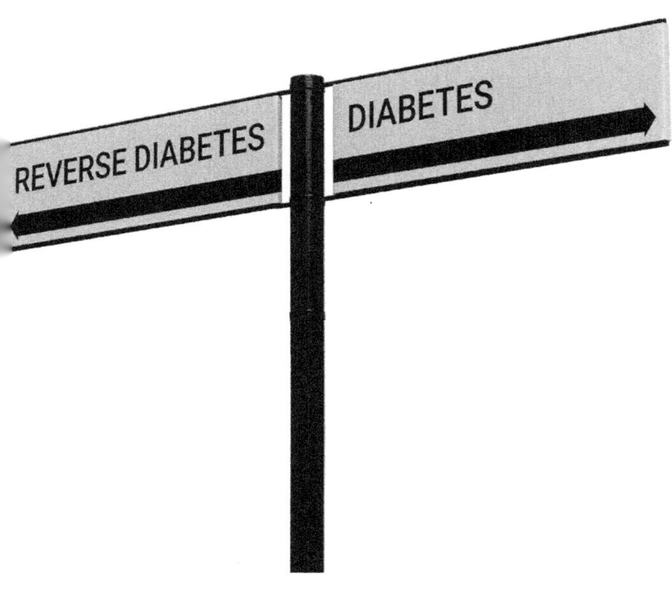

The answer to this question is yes, yes, yes! You can put type 2 diabetes in reverse. Putting something in reverse doesn't necessarily mean you go all the way back to where you started. Early on for some people, reversing diabetes to the point of remission is achievable. For others with longer standing diabetes, they will see improved blood sugar control with less medication. And, believe it or not, there are many ways to go about it. This is great news because it means there is likely a good and lasting option that will work for you.

Before we proceed, let's take a look at some figures. Type 2 diabetes is increasing at a fast rate and experts are finding that the boom is associated with global changes toward modern lifestyles. This means millions more people in recent decades are living lives that are more sedentary, urban, and offer easy access to foods high in calories, saturated fat, and sugar both day and night. It's estimated that there are 425 million people with diabetes on the planet today and that rate is expected to grow to 629 million by 2045. That's a mind-boggling number of people — almost twice the U.S. population!

The bright spot in all of this is that you don't have to become or remain one of the 425 million. Research has shown that, while unhealthy lifestyles contribute to type 2 diabetes, the opposite is also true. Healthy lifestyles can help prevent and even treat this debilitating disease. And even though type 2 diabetes is a lifelong condition once you have it, positive changes to your diet can help you reach and maintain normal blood sugar levels. How much you can improve really depends on your own individual genetics and how long you have had diabetes.

At the very least, you can make changes today to stall type 2 diabetes progression. At the very most, you may find yourself in the same happy place as many of my clients who have worked their way back to consistent, normal blood sugar levels either without medication or with reduced dosages. Now is a good time for me to introduce you to Norm.

Norm is a software executive – a witty, energetic, full of life gentleman who enjoyed mountaineering, among other activities. For the past few years, however, his energy had decreased and he'd been feeling run down.

He came to me with high blood pressure, type 2 diabetes, high cholesterol, gout, and a history of kidney cancer (one kidney had been removed). He already had a Freestyle Libre (continuous glucose monitor/CGM) and was taking multiple medications and supplements.

Norm was a grazer, that is, he usually didn't eat breakfast or lunch, but would typically start eating when he got home from work right up until bedtime. His last A1c value was high – 8.5%. His vitamin D level was low, which can impact blood sugar control.

Norm started our initial session by telling me he hadn't felt hunger in a long time; he just felt "blah." He would often eat crackers and cheese because it was easy and, if he bought a bag of chips, he could easily eat the whole bag in one sitting. He would typically drink 6–8 diet sodas a day to keep his energy level up but had recently cut back to 2 per day.

What Norm hadn't shared when we first met was that he was an amazing cook. He then started a photo food journal for me. The quality of food he prepared, as well as the presentation, was remarkable and mouthwatering.

Here was my general advice to Norm to help him get his blood sugar down in the beginning:

1. Eat an early dinner between 5–6pm. It's okay to snack on something like 2 oz. of protein or a handful of almonds when hungry.

2. Priorities: Eat 2 cups of leafy greens per day, 2 cups of sulfur-rich vegetables, or 2-3 cups of brightly colored vegetables and fruits. Then eat protein such as wild caught salmon, halibut, cod, grass-fed beef, or organic chicken.

3. Make 35g of fiber per day a goal. If eating pasta, try Banza brand made from chickpeas, or Tolerant brand made from lentils. Both of these are much higher in fiber than refined white pasta.

4. Avoid watching media while eating; try to eat meals at your table.

5. Do 15 minutes on the cardio machine each night before dinner.

Norm had to pick one or two main goals to focus on. He chose to work on vegetables first (which also helped with the fiber goal). He held off on exercise for the first month. He attempted it a few times but it's easy to get overwhelmed with all the other life changes.

He began taking vitamin D as well as magnesium glycinate and saw an immediate drop in his fasting blood sugar.

After Norm's first two weeks of ditching the chips and crackers and incorporating some vegetables and high-quality protein, he had already lost 6 pounds! And that was before he jumped on the exercise train - which took some convincing. Norm used his CGM to quickly discover which foods worked for him and which did not. He loved high-fiber whole grain English muffins but, every time he ate them, his sugar jumped much higher than he liked. Eventually he decided they weren't worth the sugar spike.

He eventually hit a rough patch and became very frustrated that he was seeing only minimal improvement. Let's be honest here - Norm was doing great. He was consistently losing 2 pounds a week, had overhauled his diet and had seen his average blood sugar drop from the 220s down to the 160s. He still had some work to do but his progress thus far was fantastic.

Eventually, we revisited the topics of sleep, stress, and movement – all of which impacted him. Norm's sleep wasn't great, he had a good deal of stress at work, and his type of work required him to be sedentary at his desk all day long. He finally committed to 5 minutes of exercise after dinner – a good place for him to start.

He found that evening was not the best time for him to exercise so he started working it in after lunch. I got a message from him one day in which he said, "I can't believe how much my blood sugar drops after exercise. It's fascinating – almost 40 points every time." The 40-point drop was after 25 minutes of exercise. Initially he started with 5 minutes after lunch, then went up to 20 minutes, 25 minutes, then 30+ minutes. And he did it every day just as he would take his medicine. His exuberance led him to increase the level on his elliptical machine. His average blood sugar was now in the 120s and his estimated average glucose on his Libre was 6.2%. Norm had lost 32 pounds and counting.

He stopped eating processed food that did not serve him well. He increased his vegetable intake, started a daily exercise routine and was able to stop his diabetes medications. He told me his next goal was to get his A1c under 6% (which he eventually achieved) and to visit Alaska to kill a 1200 pound bear with a pocket knife while reeling in a 300 pound halibut. Norm has lofty goals but his motivation was clear.

Here's what Norm wanted me to share with you:

- The magnesium was very helpful to control the morning highs.
- He liked the accountability of a photo food log. This was also helpful when looking at CGM reports to see what foods affected his blood sugar the most.
- Get creative with food choices and try things you normally wouldn't.
- Drink lots of water.
- Use the CGM to check-in with your blood sugar hourly.

Everyone's diabetes is slightly different. Having an understanding of why that is true can give you better insight on what your approach should be, as well as expected outcomes.

Type 2 diabetes is a disruption of many different systems in the body and it happens over the course of years. During these years of disruption and break down in the systems, many people may receive a diagnosis of prediabetes. This might seem boring and not very serious, but it's important to understand all the disruptions in the body that can lead to the development of type 2 diabetes. Perhaps the following will help you understand more about your diagnosis.

Genetics

Let's put the blame on mom, dad, and everyone who came before in your gene pool. Your genetics play an important role, so while you may be working hard at the gym and doing your best with food, you ended up developing diabetes anyway. You're left wondering why your friends who don't participate in any activities and eat whatever they want have no blood sugar issues at all. One simple answer here is it could be genetics. Some of us get the top-of-the-line genes while others may have been short-changed. We have to acknowledge this because, if we don't, we could very easily get discouraged by the things we can't control. Regardless, in this book we will focus on what we CAN control - which is a lot. So sit back, read on and get ready to put diabetes in reverse.

Beta Cells

Beta cell function ... say what? There are cells in your pancreas called "beta cells" and they make hormones. The one we will focus on here is called "insulin."

Remember earlier when we talked about the stubborn cells in the body becoming insulin resistant? Well, insulin resistance assists in the demise of beta cells in type 2 diabetes because glucose levels start to rise. Many people have lost over half of their beta cell function by the time they are diagnosed with diabetes. When blood sugar levels start to go higher, the pancreas has to work harder. This is why your food choices are so important. If you don't have a variety of food options on your plate and it's heavy on carbohydrates (particularly the low-fiber ones), your pancreas can become overworked.

Have you ever worked hard on a project for so long that you just became exhausted and couldn't do it anymore? This is a little like what happens to the beta cells. They are required to ramp up production of insulin because the sugar in the blood is increasing, but the cells are being resistant so the pancreas is working even harder to regulate blood sugar. When you have to work too hard for too long, productivity can decrease. The same principle applies to beta cells.

Taking care of the beta cells is important — so we need to preserve, conserve and even regenerate them. When the blood sugar is elevated, the body's ability to regenerate the cells is stunted. Researchers are looking for ways to regenerate beta cells, as this could be a cure for diabetes (type 1 and type 2). One of the best ways to conserve and preserve beta cells is to catch rising blood sugar early and not let it get out of control (sometimes this is easier said than done). The most unfortunate part of all of this is that there can be a 50% beta cell function loss — or higher — before most people are even diagnosed with type 2 diabetes.

Incretin Hormones

There are two main incretin hormones (made in the gut to help decrease blood sugar levels). Glucagon-like Peptide 1 (GLP-1) helps regulate your appetite, especially after eating. It also helps enhance insulin production. GLP-1 helps your body to slow down how quickly food is emptied from the gut. It helps tell your brain when you've had enough and it helps your pancreas release the right amount of insulin.

The other incretin hormone worth mentioning is glucose-dependent insulinotropic peptide (GIP). This hormone is produced in the small intestine after we eat. Its main action is to encourage the release of insulin into the bloodstream to control blood sugar. This function is lost in people with type 2 diabetes. It has been shown however, that after being given GLP-1, the ability to secrete insulin can be restored. So now we have an injectable form of this hormone that some people take to help manage their diabetes.

Insulin Resistance

In prediabetes and diabetes, the cells are being stubborn (insulin resistance). They are not letting the sugar enter into the cell, particularly after eating a meal with carbohydrates, causing the blood sugar to rise higher than normal. This is also usually the culprit of post-meal sleepiness. We just consumed energy but our body isn't able to use it because it's not getting into the cells properly.

Liver

Cue a spotlight on the liver as it's one of the busiest organs in the body. Its role in diabetes is important because the liver is supposed to store up sugar (prompted by insulin release from the pancreas) after we eat. It's basically a storage unit for glucose in case we run low. We run into problems if the body is having trouble making insulin (as we discussed previously regarding beta cell loss). The liver relies on insulin to signal it to stop or start producing sugar. So if there is not a lot of insulin, the liver thinks the body needs more sugar and it starts dumping sugar into the blood (even when it's not supposed to). It is making more glucose than necessary while we are in a resting state. The body has trouble shutting down this production, often contributing to a higher blood sugar after we have gone without food for a long period, such as after sleep. This is frequently the reason some people complain about a higher blood sugar when they wake up in the morning.

High Levels of Fat in the Blood

When we eat and digest our food, free fatty acids are released into the bloodstream. When we have high levels of free fatty acids in the blood, it can inhibit the body's ability to produce insulin. When the body can't make insulin as well, blood sugar will increase. It's important to eat the right kinds of fat and we will talk about that later. All fats are not created equal.

Excess Storage

A clinical term for excess storage of fuel leading to an increased body weight is "obesity." Obesity is a disease state that can lead to increased insulin resistance. It is also a complicated disease that we won't explore in this book. However, it is a disease just as diabetes is. When obesity is coupled with other diseases, such as high levels of fat in the blood, this can lead to chronic inflammation and can affect several systems in the body. When someone has obesity, it is highly likely that they have intestinal permeability (also known as leaky gut). By decreasing inflammation and addressing leaky gut, obesity can begin to be resolved.

Note: Obesity is not just about calories in, calories out, and moving more. It's just not that simple. Oversimplifying the disease of obesity has led to a weight-based stigma and discrimination. This increases susceptibility to psychological distress that may further contribute to poor health.

Lack of Movement

When we find ourselves less physically active, perhaps due to a lack of time or to an injury, our bodies require less energy to function. Often as we slow down, we don't necessarily decrease our fuel (food) and this can be one contributing factor to weight gain, blood pressure, blood sugar, and blood cholesterol issues. Exercise is an important tool to manage or reverse diabetes. One-hundred fifty minutes a week is recommended as a maintenance dose of exercise to keep our bodies healthy and responsive to insulin the body makes. Exercise benefits our gut bacteria and helps to improve our gut lining as well.

High Levels of Sugar in the Blood

When you have insulin resistance and decreased insulin production, over time, this can lead to very high levels of glucose in the bloodstream referred to as "glucotoxicity." Long-term exposure to high blood sugar levels also contributes to decreased insulin output. It's as though the body becomes overwhelmed and, instead of ramping up production to fix the problem, the beta cells shut down and this vicious cycle continues. Sometimes in this case, when blood sugar levels go up into the 200mg/dl+ range consistently, a shot of insulin or another diabetes medication might be necessary to help improve insulin sensitivity and help clear some of the sugar in the blood.

Note: Medication can be a temporary aid depending on where you are in the diabetes progression. I have seen many people use insulin for a month or two to help out their pancreas and then they are able to stop and use a pill, food, and/or movement to manage their blood sugar.

Gut Bacteria

There are trillions of gut bacteria that live in the body. The body acts as a vehicle for these microbes. The gut microbiome is the set of genes in our gastrointestinal tract. It has 3 million genes, which is considerably larger than our human genome.

Gut bacteria play an important role in diabetes development as well as blood sugar control. By feeding your gut bacteria sufficient fiber, you help the good bacteria flourish which can be a key factor in regulating blood glucose.

The intestinal lining of the gut should be intact. Certain foods can loosen the tight junctions of the intestinal wall. According to a review in the journal, ***Nutrition Research***, bacteria and bacterial fragments cross the intestinal barrier and can start an inflammatory process that can prevent insulin from working properly.

So, did diabetes start because of genetics, or beta cells, or what? Nope, I saved the best for last. Often, the root cause of diabetes being triggered into action is dysbiosis (imbalance of gut bacteria), inflammation, and intestinal permeability. We will spend a lot of time talking about the 5 steps to healing which will help with shifting diabetes into reverse. But first — I bet you were wondering — can't I just take a pill?

CHAPTER 3

Can't I Just Take Pills?

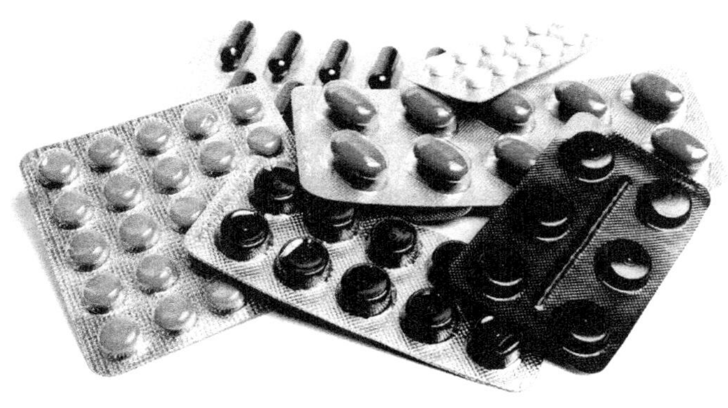

Well, yes, technically you could just take pills. Providers prescribe pills every day for diabetes. The thing is though that diabetes is different. Diabetes is a progressive disease and, if you only take pills and do nothing else, it's harder to slow its progression or reverse it. If you approach diabetes from several angles, the chance of taming it is far better.

Many people take their diabetes pills, do nothing else, and they're fine ... for awhile. Eventually the doctor visit will come whereupon they find out their A1c is slowly creeping up, or they start feeling more tired than usual, or start experiencing pain or tingling in their feet. Diabetes is a silent disease. A person might accept some of the problems it causes as a consequence of growing older, but many complications of diabetes can be slowed or prevented. Using only one of the tools in your toolbox, however, isn't going to cut it.

Clients often tell me they want to reduce their diabetes medications for various reasons. Some complain about the cost, some don't like the side effects, and for others, it's as simple as not liking swallowing pills. In no way do I want to demonize medications, as some people truly need them, depending on where they are in the diabetes journey. But what if there was a way to come off of some of the medications or postpone the need for as long as possible? What if there were other treatments?

Well, there are! That's why you chose to pick up this book. I promise we will get to all the treatments, but let's start by taking a look at some of the classes of diabetes medications. It's good to know what you are taking and how it works in your body. This will help you if you are currently on medications or if you think you may need them down the road.

Some people use diabetes medications right after diagnosis to get their blood sugar under control quickly, then come off over time. Others get diagnosed with diabetes early on and control it with other means. Years down the road, some find medications are helpful in maintaining good blood sugar control and preventing complications. Using medications does not mean you have failed. You cannot control everything, such as genetics, as we discussed earlier.

Remember, medications need to be in your toolbox – just in case. You will use some tools more than others and will probably discover a favorite tool which provides good outcomes. We will fill up your toolbox and you will get to choose what you like best and what helps you the most.

Let's talk about medications. We have come a long way in understanding and treating diabetes, and we have a lot of new and improved medications that are much better than some of the old ones. You need to be able to make educated decisions, along with your healthcare provider, about the best medication options for you – if you indeed need them at some point.

My preferred medications for clients:

I do not receive any financial support from any of these companies. I just have strong opinions about which medications I prefer for my clients. Medications are constantly changing and new ones are being added, so here are some of the general ones that have been around for a few years or longer.

TYPES OF MEDICATIONS	**SGLT2 Inhibitors** Canagliflozin/Invokana Dapagliflozin/Farxiga Empagliflozin/Jardiance Ertugliflozin/Steglatro
WHERETHEYWORK IN THE BODY	Keeps your kidneys from reabsorbing some of the sugar and then excreting it. Because calories get excreted, there is a potential for weight loss.
PROS	Does not cause weight gain, can help with weight loss and high blood pressure, and may reduce cardiovascular disease (CVD) risk.
CONS	Because you are excreting extra sugar, if you are prone to yeast infections or urinary tract infections, this can increase your risk of getting one. This is not a great medication if your blood sugar is really high; it will lower A1c about .5% to 1%.
WHY I LIKE THEM AND IMPORTANT NOTES	Can support weight maintenance or weight loss with minimal side effects. Be sure to stay hydrated while on this medication. There is usually little to no chance of hypoglycemia.

TYPES OF MEDICATIONS	**DPP IV inhibitor** Alogliptin/Nesina Linagliptin/Tradjenta Saxagliptin/Onglyza Sitagliptin/Januvia Vildagliptin/Galvus (not approved in US yet)	**Biguanides** Metformin/Glucophage
WHERE THEY WORK IN THE BODY	Helps keep your GLP1 hormone around longer to get the benefits of fullness, decreased appetite.	Changes the gut microbiota and liver cells
PROS	Does not cause weight gain; can help with weight loss	Very effective at lowering blood sugar, may have positive impact on gut bacteria, inexpensive, and does not cause weight gain, may even cause weight loss. Can increase good bacteria like Akkermansia, and increases butyrate, which is good for gut health
CONS	Alone, this medication will only reduce A1c level by about 0.6–0.8%. This is for people who just need a little help getting their sugar down.	Many people get stomach distress/ diarrhea, so extended release formula is best. In 2020, there were recalls related to a cancer-causing substance, NDMA. Pills are large. Metformin can cause a Vitamin B12 deficiency, so it may be necessary to supplement with 1,000-2000mcg B12 daily.
WHY I LIKE THEM AND IMPORTANT NOTES	Supports weight maintenance or weight loss with minimal side effects. Be sure to stay hydrated while on this medication. Little to no chance of hypoglycemia.	Reduces A1c 1%-2 %. This is a very effective tool to get your blood sugar down quickly if you are newly diagnosed. One of the best medications we have for diabetes, if tolerated.

GLP1 Receptor Agonist (injectable)	**Insulin (injectable or inhaled)**
*Albiglutide/Tanzeum *Dulaglutide/Trulicity Exenatide/Byetta (twice a day) *Extended-release exenatide/Bydureon Liraglutide/Victoza Lixisenatide/Adlyxin *Semaglutide/Ozempic Semaglutide/Rybelsus (oral pill, not injection) *These injections are given weekly.	Long Acting/Ultra Long Acting Glargine/Lantus or Basaglar, lasts up to 24 hours. Degludec/Tresiba, lasts up to 42 hours. Detemir/Levemir, lasts 18 to 23 hours. Glargine/Toujeo, lasts more than 24 hours. Degludec/Tresiba, lasts up to 42 hours. Fast and Rapid Acting / Inhalable Aspart/Novolog, Fiasp (faster) Glulisine/Apidra Lispro/Humalog Afrezza (inhaled insulin)
Increases insulin output while telling your body not to make sugar, but only when glucose levels are elevated. Very smart! It also slows food from entering into your blood as quickly so you feel full, and there is less of a spike in blood sugar after you eat.	Injecting or inhaling insulin is like sending in reinforcements for your pancreas. Insulin is a hormone that your body makes, and the key that unlocks cells so glucose (sugar) can enter. Insulin regulates sugar in the body.
Does not cause weight gain, and many see weight loss. Also beneficial for high blood pressure and reducing CVD. Shown to reduce A1C by ~0.8%-1.6%. This works great for people who spike after meals; it's a nice alternative to mealtime insulin in type 2 diabetes.	If you are newly diagnosed and your blood sugar has been in the 300s, and your A1c is >9%, taking some long-acting insulin for a month or two might help your pancreas and stop the glucose toxicity/ insulin resistance cycle. Contrary to popular belief, once you start insulin, it doesn't mean you are on it for life. It's just a tool and an amazing one at that.
If you have had pancreatitis or have very high triglycerides, such as over 500, this is not the best medication for you. Also, people with a history of gallbladder issues should be cautious with this medication. It can cause nausea, gastrointestinal (GI) upset, and heartburn in some. It's important to start at a very low dose to see if you tolerate it. More expensive than other meds.	Insulin is a fat-storing hormone. So if you are on insulin for the long-haul, you HAVE to change your food intake or you will gain weight. Low glycemic eating works very well for people on insulin. You are at risk for hypoglycemia if you take insulin. Know the signs, symptoms, and how to treat.
Supports weight loss, minimal side effects. Be sure to stay hydrated while on this medication and eat mindfully. Focus on eating the most nutritious foods first as your intake may be reduced drastically and you don't want to become malnourished. Little to no chance of hypoglycemia.	Insulin is a great way to get blood sugar back on track. If you are newly diagnosed with type 2 diabetes and your blood sugar has been in the 300s, and/or your A1c is >10%, taking long-acting insulin for a month or two might help your pancreas and stop glucose toxicity/ insulin resistance cycle.

*Amylin is not mentioned. While it's a great medication, it is used mainly in type 1 diabetes (has to be injected before each meal), and we have once-weekly GLP-1 that gives great results, particularly in type 2 diabetes.

My least favorite medications for clients:

TYPE OF ME DICATION	WHERE THEY WORK	PROS	CONS
Sulfonylureas	Tells the pancreas to make more insulin, "exhausting" it	Lowers blood sugar quickly, inexpensive	Weight gain, hypoglycemia, wears out the beta cells
Meglitinides Repaglinide/ Prandin Nateglinide/Starlix	Tells the pancreas to make more insulin	Help post-meal blood sugar spike	Weight gain, hypoglycemia, have to take at each meal (increases chances of forgetting medication)
Alpha Glucosidase Inhibitors Acarbose/Precose Miglitol/Glyset	Works in the stomach to delay the digestion of carbohydrate and intestinal absorption of glucose	Feel fuller longer, lower post-meal blood sugar, lowers HbA1c by 0.5%-1.0%	Have to take before each meal (possibility of forgetting), GI upset/ gas
TZD/PPARy agonists (Thiazolidinediones) Pioglitazone/Actos Rosiglitazone/Avandia	Causes the body to produce new fat cells that are more sensitive to insulin- a round-about way of making your insulin resistance decrease	Improves insulin sensitivity	Weight gain, edema (fluid retention), increased risk of heart failure, increased bone fracture risk

*There are also Bile Acid Sequestrants and Dopamine 2 Agonists but they are not worth mentioning as I rarely see them used. We have newer, more targeted, better options now.

The Impact of Medications on the Wallet

From 2012 to 2017, the total costs of diagnosed diabetes increased by 26%. The American Diabetes Association estimates the total costs of diabetes have risen to $327 billion in 2017 from $245 billion in 2012. The American Diabetes Association also states that people with diabetes incur average medical costs of $16,752 per year and $9,601 is attributed to diabetes.

This is serious! Think of all the things you could do and places you could go if you had an extra $9,000 in your pocket. Some medications have been around longer than others, and therefore, they are a bit cheaper. Regardless, I think we can all agree that less is more when it comes to medications. No matter how long you've had diabetes, there are always ways to reduce your medication needs. It's time now for you to meet Greg.

Greg had just retired a few years ago and had been struggling with diabetes and his weight for a long time. Several years prior, he had gastric bypass surgery which really helped him. He lost a significant amount of weight and was able to come off of his insulin immediately after surgery. Fast forward to retirement and the weight started creeping back up. He was back on insulin and he also started smoking again, but was using Chantix to quit. He was on three different diabetes medications. His A1c was elevated: 7.8%.

When he came to me, he had slipped back into some bad habits. He still couldn't eat very much food at one time because of his gastric bypass surgery, but often his choices were not filled with optimal nutrition. He had been under a lot of stress for many years with his job and, although retirement had brought him some much needed peace, he continued to do some contract work and stress was still a factor. His wife walks nearly every day so he mentioned he would resume joining her.

He had the following goals:

- Quit smoking permanently
- Exercise daily
- Eat a much healthier diet – but was not sure what that meant
- Get his A1C below 7 and keep it there
- Reduce or eliminate as much medication as possible – in particular, the insulin shots

We worked together to create his "why" statement – which you did as well in Chapter 1. This is what he came up with: I want a high-quality life to enjoy my family, and be functional and present for them. I know that food and exercise are good medicines and I want to give them a chance to work for me, allowing for less insulin and pills.

I reminded him that he always has choices and to pause and choose options that align with the goals that have been set. It's important to remind yourself of your goals each day.

He would often snack before bed to change the taste in his mouth. His late night snacks were usually trigger foods. Trigger foods are those you typically crave when you're not hungry and struggle to stop once you start eating them. Having trigger foods nearby can exhaust willpower and set a person up for failure.

We also revisited his "why" as well as his goals to see if the choice to eat late at night aligned with what he was trying to accomplish. He concluded that it did not.

Bottomline:

Really understand why you make the food choices you make. This is not about good and bad foods; it's not about deprivation. It's about making decisions about food that will help you reach your health goals.

For the first week he chose the following goals:

1. Daily exercise for 10–40 minutes.

2. Avoid snacking while watching TV. Mindless eating leads to an increased need for diabetes medications. Use food to heal and not as a recreational drug. If you need to eat due to hunger, eat on a plate or bowl at the kitchen table. If it's only about changing the taste in your mouth, try brushing your teeth or drinking an herbal flavored, unsweetened tea.

3. If you have an ongoing metallic taste, that needs to be explored further with your healthcare provider, as the cause could be medication or a vitamin.

Note: When desserts are available, make sure they are worth choosing. They should be good quality, a high priority and worthy of your tastebuds.

After 3 weeks, Greg's total insulin needs dropped from 64 units per day to 20 units. Calculated, healthier food choices were helping him feel better along with his daily exercise.

Eventually his A1c dropped to 7%. Greg was now off his insulin, although his metformin dose was increased. Greg's A1c is now less than 6%. He is still off insulin and he's feeling great. Greg is no different than you or anyone else. If he can do it, so can you.

What if we started thinking about food and activity as medicine as well?

All carbohydrates come from the earth — whether picked from the ground like grains, or picked from a tree like some fruits. They contain important nutrients including vitamins, minerals, fiber and antioxidants. How we prepare those carbohydrates, the amount we eat at one time, and what time of day we eat them can impact blood sugar levels. If you consume a lot of carbohydrates at once when you have diabetes, it can challenge your body's ability to respond appropriately. We will dive deeper into carbohydrates in a little bit.

What you need to know now is that people with type 2 diabetes cannot process a lot of sugar (carbohydrate) at one time and, therefore, have trouble clearing it out of the blood. High blood sugar leaves blood thick and syrupy with sugar and, as a result, the person feels like it's time for a nap. Not to mention the wear and tear on your heart as it has to pump that thick syrupy blood throughout the body.

If carbohydrates are eaten in smaller doses throughout the day, the body has more time to process them and energy remains stable. The same concept applies to protein and fat. Reasonable amounts of fat and protein at mealtime will help with feeling full and satisfied until your next meal. Vegetables are an excellent remedy to stop sugar cravings while enabling the good bacteria in our gut to thrive. They also provide bulk and make us feel full.

Finally, besides insulin, I don't know of a better medicine than movement. Greg showed us the power of exercise. Many of my clients report a big drop in blood sugar with less than 30 minutes of moderate activity, which is an example of exercise as medicine. The rate at which blood sugar drops from exercise can depend on a lot. These factors include your blood sugar level before you started, stress level, medications you take, as well as the intensity, type and duration of exercise.

Several of my clients with type 2 diabetes have been able to reduce their dose or completely stop their insulin. Each time exercise was a key component.

Meet Monica. Monica is in her 30s, has a demanding job and is a woman of faith. She had been praying for a long time that she would be able to get off of insulin.

If you asked Monica why it is important to exercise and choose healthy food, she would tell you – to stay off insulin and to be able to start a family. Monica loves dessert, however, just like many of us.

When Monica describes her "future self", she projects that she will be living in Arizona or Texas near her relatives, will walk and hike everyday with her future children, and will go to the gym 2-3 times per week. She enjoys cooking healthy meals with her family and healthy eating in general. She sees herself working from home part-time and starting a family business with her sister.

When I first met her, Monica was taking long-acting and rapid-acting insulin. She had been diagnosed with polycystic ovarian syndrome (PCOS) and then eventually diabetes. She was very clear and upfront that she was not interested in an insulin pump or a continuous glucose monitor. She typically checked her sugar at least 4–6 times a day.

We asked Monica's healthcare provider to start her on metformin so we could increase her sensitivity to the insulin she was getting and address her PCOS. There are other ways to address PCOS as well, but this was the best fit for her at this time. We were able to decrease her insulin dose right away. In the meantime, she started eating more mindfully. She was cutting back on nighttime eating and incorporating more vegetables into her meals while still enjoying some, but fewer,

> *Note about insulin: When most people think about units of insulin, they tend to think about U-100 insulin because that was all we had for many years. But there are different "power levels" of insulin. When insulin says U-200 on the vial, it means it's twice as powerful. So if someone is taking 20 units of U-200 insulin, it's the same as taking 40 units of U-100.*

desserts. She had a highly stressful job and a very busy life. She exercised when she could, but struggled with consistency. Every time she did exercise, however, she noted how much better she felt mentally and physically.

To add more into the mix, she bought a new place to live. As she started packing up and moving, life got very hectic and she forgot to refill her insulin, missing a day or two of her medicine. During this move which demanded a high level of energy and activity, she was also checking her blood sugar more often. It was then that she noticed that it was better than when she had been taking insulin. This was the "why" she had been dreaming of. She had been working very hard on a lifestyle of changes to try to get off insulin but had not yet experienced what it could be like and if it would really work.

This was a turning point for Monica. She had missed a few days of insulin while she was vigorously active during her move. She realized that her body could function in a way that would give her a chance to discontinue taking insulin. Her "why" just got stronger. Not only did she experience the change for a few days, she was now motivated to keep on exercising. To this day, she has not needed to resume taking insulin. Her average blood sugar ranges from 130–155 with her CGM and she can see how food is affecting her. Although she still struggles to keep work life, personal life, classes, exercise and food in harmony — she is determined to continue a lifestyle that does not require insulin.

I also want to mention that when Monica was diagnosed with diabetes, she was given some pills to bring her high blood sugar levels down. A week later, she went into Diabetic Ketoacidosis (DKA). DKA is a serious condition when your cells can't get the glucose they need and your body begins to burn fat for fuel. Ketones are produced and start to build up in the blood. This is different from "ketosis" in people doing the keto diet. DKA is when blood sugar levels are high and ketones are high. This led her healthcare providers to believe she had type 1 diabetes and that was her original diagnosis. We now know, that is not the case.

During those few days when Monica missed her medicine, she realized that her initial diagnosis may have been wrong. Someone who has type 1 diabetes cannot go without insulin for an extended period of time without major repercussions.

NOTE: Please do not stop taking the medications your doctor has prescribed!

There is a methodical and safe way to go about change, so don't feel the need to rush. By taking it step-by-step along with your healthcare provider, you can begin to reverse your diabetes. People who rush to get off their medication are sometimes disappointed. Think of medications as a tool, if you stop using that tool too soon, it makes it very hard to get to the end of the "project." The key in all of this is to first get your blood sugar into target range with the tools that you have. Then, as you slowly start using food and activity to manipulate your blood sugar, your body will begin to respond more effectively and efficiently to those approaches, and your medication can start to be reduced. Always do this with the help of your provider.

As you begin this process, continue to evaluate everything. Just as you would evaluate a new medication that made you feel sick, tell your doctor about any effects you notice with food and exercise. The changes you make should feel good, be easy, manageable and sustainable day-after-day. Jump-starting too many changes at once in diet or exercise can set you up for failure, as those things may not necessarily feel right. You might see great results with your blood sugar right away, but what good is it if it doesn't last?

Walking, biking, dancing or any activity that sounds appealing is the best medicine. Start with a few minutes after eating and see what happens. This is when your blood sugar meter or continuous glucose monitor can earn its keep.

Paired Testing

The Paired Testing technique will give you the most feedback about your food, activity and how it affects you. One way is to check your sugar right before a meal and then 2 hours after to see how well your body processed the carbohydrates. On a different day, you could check your sugar before you eat, then do your movement of choice for at least 10–15 minutes and again see what your blood sugar is 2 hours after. Start learning what foods are your best medicine and what dose of movement you need to get the results you want. The goal is to have a 30–50 mg/dl increase in blood sugar (or less) from before a meal to 2 hours after you eat.

Note about mealtime insulin: If you are on mealtime insulin and your blood sugar does not go up at least 30 mg/dl, consider reducing your mealtime insulin dose. Rapid-acting mealtime-insulin hangs around in your body for 3-6 hours and it peaks at 1.5 to 2 hours. So if your blood sugar barely rises after you eat and you still have a couple hours of active insulin in your body, you are at high risk of getting low blood sugar in the next couple hours. Low blood sugar can make you shaky, dizzy, sweaty, incoherent, and possibly lead to unconsciousness. You should treat low blood sugar with a quick acting carbohydrate such as 4 ounces of juice. Chocolate candy bars are not an ideal blood sugar treatment since anything with higher fat content can slow the sugar's entry into your bloodstream. You may find a way to work chocolate into your meal plan if you love it but, when your blood sugar is low, quick acting sugar is best.

Alright, it's finally time. Let's begin to discuss the basics of meal planning to reverse diabetes. We will eventually go deeper than the basics that follow, but we have to start somewhere.

The Basics of Meal Planning

STEP 1: Non-starchy Vegetables

The non-starchy vegetables group comes first for a reason. It's the most important group because it has the ability to help lower blood sugar, heal inflammation, feed your good gut bacteria and has the most curative properties of all the food groups. The proper serving of non-starchy vegetables would fit in both hands if you cupped them together. They should cover half your plate. It could be a salad (in a bowl) plus another vegetable or two, such as steamed broccoli, broiled brussels sprouts, asparagus, etc. There are dozens of vegetable choices so pick the ones that taste best to you and your family. Vegetables are anti-inflammatory and promote healing. We want to make sure we get plenty of them.

SOME EXAMPLES OF NON-STARCHY VEGETABLES:

Artichoke, asparagus, bok choy, green beans, broccoli, cabbage, carrots, cauliflower, celery, cucumber, green beans, leafy greens (kale, spinach, arugula, etc), leeks, mushrooms, okra, onions, peppers, tomatoes, and zucchini

STEP 2: Carbohydrates (Fiber)

One-quarter of your plate can include starchy vegetables (more or less depending on how active you are). Sweet potatoes, black beans, lentils, chickpea pasta, brown rice, quinoa or any ancient grains are examples. A good rule of thumb is anything that grows from the ground would fit here, but what's important is it needs to be high in fiber content. If you are low on pantry goods, you could even substitute or add a little fruit here if you wanted. Some people have issues with certain grains and beans, so pay close attention to how your body responds to these foods. If you have gas or bloating after a meal, it's likely one of these could be the culprit. If you start feeling sleepy after a meal, this is the group you should examine further. Sometimes introducing small amounts of these high fiber foods and gradually building up works well to manage the gas or bloating.

STEP 3: Protein

Finally, choose a protein. This can include fish, chicken, pork, beef, wild game, tofu or another protein. When choosing protein from a land animal, those that are wild or grass-fed are typically best. Fish is at the top of the list for anti-inflammatory proteins, so that's a good option to choose at least 2–3 times a week. Fish provides vitamin D and omega 3 fatty acids that help decrease inflammation.

Aim for about 3 to 6 ounces of protein at a meal. A general rule of thumb, if you will, is using the palm of your hand and the thickness of your pinky as a reference in determining the amount you should eat. Note that this is a general statement and, therefore, not individualized to you personally. Your choice of protein will cover the other quarter of your plate. There will be exceptions when it comes to the amount and, in the coming chapters, more details will be provided about the quality and quantity of the foods you choose.

The last ingredient in this meal preparation is permission to enjoy your meal, knowing there will be no guilt or regret afterward. If you follow this formula, you can choose foods which you and your family like while still maintaining your weight, your health and feelings of being satisfied rather than deprived. I constantly hear people judging themselves regarding meals. Stop doing that! Own what you eat and enjoy it. Be mindful of your choices yet enjoy the experience of eating.

Over time, you will notice which foods your body responds to best. I encourage you to pay attention to that instead of following a "diet" with guidelines and restrictions. The goal here is to find something you can live with and know that not every cookie-cutter diet plan works for everyone. It feels good to be in charge of your food choices and not live by rules set by other people.

This basic concept of meal planning is called the plate method — with a few tweaks. It's a nice method to use when trying to plan a meal or while at a gathering or restaurant and filling your plate.

CHAPTER 4

Herbs and Supplements for Diabetes

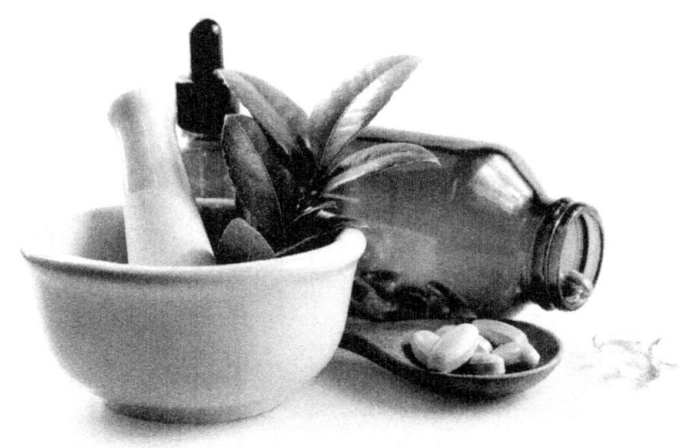

At this point, we have talked about medications and touched briefly on food and exercise — but what about supplements? This is one of the questions I get asked most frequently.

It's important to address supplements here because sometimes they are viewed as more desirable than medications. Some supplements can help, while others may be a waste of money.

We should try to get as many of our daily vitamins and nutrients from food as possible, but due to soil quality, growing and picking practices, sometimes food quality is compromised and leaves us with a deficiency. By no means should you give up on fruits and vegetables. This just lends to the case for eating more. Many supplements for diabetes are meant to help repair and restore the body. Ideally, once you've removed the food that is not serving your body, or increased a low micronutrient level, your gut can begin to repair and the inflammation starts to decrease. This is where supplements may come in handy.

It is important to choose high quality pharmaceutical grade supplements that have undergone testing. Many supplements at your local drug store will not necessarily meet those requirements. I highly recommend working with a registered dietitian who specializes in integrative functional nutrition or an integrative functional provider/naturopath to help you make the best choices. Just because you can purchase herbs and supplements without a prescription does not necessarily mean you should. There can be side effects and supplement/medication interactions. Please do your homework first and consult with a team of professionals to assist you.

Vitamin D

Vitamin D is one of the most common vitamin deficiencies I see in diabetes. This is especially true living in Alaska where we don't get a lot of sun in the winter. Even in the summer when we have plenty of sun, it's a very short window during which our bodies can use the sun to convert it to vitamin D.

The darker your skin, the less vitamin D your body can make from the sun. Even if you live in the sunniest of places, vitamin D deficiency is still very possible. It's important to get your vitamin D levels checked. People with low vitamin D are more likely to develop diabetes.

Optimal vitamin D levels are 50–80 ng/mL. When you are within this optimal range you have a 50% reduced risk of developing breast cancer and a decreased risk of developing other cancers. When your vitamin D is under 50, you are at twice the risk of a heart attack, have an increased incidence of high blood pressure and are three times more likely to be diagnosed with multiple sclerosis. This is serious. If you are not yet convinced of the fact that food is truly medicine, read on.

When vitamin D level drops below 30, a person is at increased risk of the following: osteoporosis, poor wound healing, joint and back pain, depression, diabetes, schizophrenia, migraines, autoimmune disease, allergies, preeclampsia, and overall inflammation. Take a moment to process that. You can prevent conditions or, at the very least, decrease your risk of many of those conditions by making sure you get sufficient vitamin D. In order to achieve this, you would need to have 50 mcg of vitamin D or 2,000 IU daily from food.

In Alaska, marine mammals such as seals, whales, salmon, trout and wild birds are the best source of vitamin D. It's amazing how nature provides what you need based on where you live, especially since Alaska is low on sunshine for half the year. What does nature provide where you live?

Take it with Vitamin D with K2 – MK7(menaquinone). Vitamin K2 helps to get calcium into the bones and out of the heart, joints, and kidneys. There is also some data that menaquinones may be associated with reduced risk of type 2 diabetes.

Magnesium

Magnesium (Mg) serves an important role in more than 300 reactions in the body. Magnesium deficiency is common in type 2 diabetes. Both high blood sugar and high insulin levels increase magnesium excretion in the urine. A magnesium deficiency can make a person with diabetes less sensitive to their insulin (which means higher blood sugar) and experience increased arrhythmias, more rapid decline of renal function, and cognitive decline.

Magnesium is involved in the regulation of dopamine levels in the body. Dopamine is a neurotransmitter involved in many important processes in the body. We also need magnesium to help blood vessels relax.

Magnesium can be lost in urine due to diuretic use, leading to low magnesium levels. If you are on a diuretic, such as furosemide or hydrochlorothiazide, you are at risk of low magnesium.

Most older adults in the U.S. don't get the proper amount of magnesium in their diets. It's best to eat dark, leafy green vegetables, unrefined grains, and legumes to keep your magnesium level up. Too much magnesium from a supplement (particularly Mg oxide) can have a laxative affect. Magnesium oxide is often given for constipation, and not absorbed as well.

Bottomline:

If you are deficient in magnesium, consider magnesium glycinate. It is the one of the best forms of magnesium for people with diabetes. I recommend 400–800 mg daily. It can help improve blood sugar, reduce cravings and also help with anxiety and sleep. Remember - a blood test at the doctor's office is not an accurate detector of low magnesium; you need a micronutrient test.

Potential Supplements

Some of my favorite supplements for diabetes are:

HERB/SUPPLEMENT	HOW IT HELPS
Chromium Picolinate	Helps with glucose metabolism when combined with biotin.
Gymnema Sylvestre	Can reduce the amount of sugar absorbed by intestines and stimulate release of insulin from the pancreas; a tincture works best
Alpha Lipoic Acid	Increases insulin sensitivity by activating AMPK in skeletal muscle. This helps the body use its own insulin better; can also be beneficial for nerve damage from diabetes
Bilberry	Helps your body respond better to a meal with carbohydrates; helps with improved circulation; can be beneficial for eye health
Bitter Melon	Suppresses gluconeogenesis, which means it tells your liver to stop making excess sugar
Berberine	Improves metabolic and insulin responses, can lower blood pressure and blood cholesterol; is also an antimicrobial; great at assisting with gut dysbiosis

HERB/SUPPLEMENT	HOW IT HELPS
Vanadyl/Vanadium	Can help improve insulin sensitivity
Quercetin	Can stimulate glucose uptake; is an antioxidant; its anti-inflammatory effects may help reduce inflammation, kill cancer cells, and help prevent heart disease
Banaba	Helps the body use insulin more efficiently
Fenugreek	Improves insulin response
Stinging Nettle	May assist in delaying absorption of carbohydrates, increase insulin secretion, and make cells more sensitive to insulin
Biotin (B7)	Helps with insulin resistance, especially when paired with chromium; found in organ meats, dairy, legumes, leafy greens, nuts, and mushrooms
Cinnamon Bark	Improves insulin sensitivity; antioxidant support
CoQ10	May help with insulin resistance and lowering fasting blood glucose levels

Women who are breastfeeding or pregnant should not try any herbs without the supervision of their provider. Also, these herbs and supplements can be powerful. Just because it's a "natural" approach doesn't mean it's a free-for-all. Some herbs are not meant to be taken long-term. All of them sound amazing, so before you head to your local drug store to stock up, consider partnering with an integrative functional provider who can give you knowledgeable guidance and be part of your team. No need to go it alone.

Here are some reputable brands whose ingredients include a combination of some of the herbs listed above.

Diabenil® by Thorne®

Gluco IR by Nutri Dyn

GlucoBalance® by Biotics Research

Glycemic Manager™ by Integrative Therapeutics

Note: **The downside to using herbs is that you may end up taking 5 or more pills a day. Herbs can have interactions with other medications, so I cannot stress enough the importance of working with a practitioner. Just because there is over-the-counter access to all of these doesn't necessarily mean any**

or all is a good fit for you. Quality matters in supplements just like it does in food. Be transparent with your provider if you take supplements and always work with a knowledgeable practitioner.

Bottomline:

You need to be methodical and patient when working with herbs and supplements. Try one product at a time, measure your blood sugar, pay attention to how you feel and really understand how your body responds. We likely will never have large random clinical-controlled trials for herbs and supplements. Instead, one must use the safety data we have on some of these herbs, take a cautious approach, and really take the time to evaluate their impact. Evidence-based nutrition is not just about random clinical-controlled trials, but also about clinical experience as well. Have I mentioned the importance of having an integrative functional medicine provider, experienced in diabetes, on your team?

CHAPTER 5

Quality, Quantity and Diversity

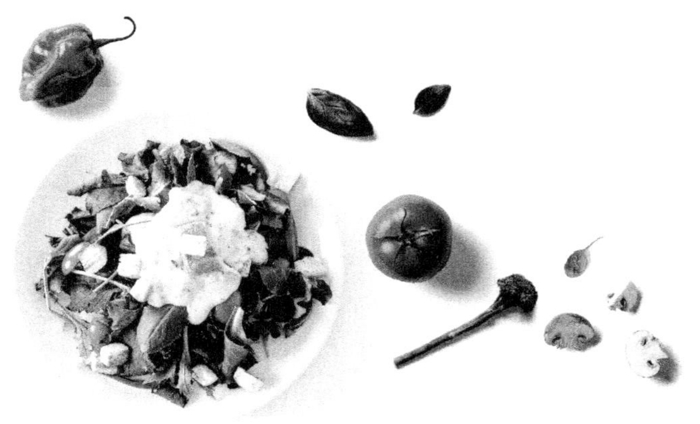

What diet works best for reversing diabetes? Answer: quality, quantity and diversity

So what eating style is best for type 2 diabetes? This is a trick question. It can be tempting to treat a disease tied to unhealthy lifestyles with the shiniest new diet trends, particularly the ones that claim to be the pinnacle of healthy living. But I hate, loathe and despise the word diet. To me "diet" means rules, restrictions, guilt and failure. Let's banish those four horsemen to the last century where they belong.

Another thing people think of when they hear "diet" is a specific (often rigid) system of eating, such as the Keto Diet, the Paleo Diet, or the Vegan Diet. While these plans work well for some people, not everyone is suited to follow, enjoy, or succeed with them. I hope you are relieved to hear this. I'm not going to tell you there is only one way to eat to improve your type 2 diabetes. The best way is the way that works for you. Allow me to explain.

When I talk about diet, what I really mean is the food that one eats in the course of a day. We could also use words like "eating style," or the types of foods you are drawn to. The term diet used this way simply refers to what you eat and does not imply restrictions. So let's go ahead and determine your diet/eating style so as to begin the process of reversing type 2 diabetes.

Grab your notebook and write down your thoughts to the following steps. It will make much more sense and become very simple when you see it in black and white.

Step 1: Pick your eating style.

Write down a list of foods that make you actually feel the best. Include the foods you enjoy and the foods that give you the most energy. Do these foods mostly grow from plants and trees or do these foods walk and swim before you eat them? Great! On to the next step.

Step 2: Determine how you will get your fiber.

Are you drawn to nuts, seeds, leafy greens, vegetables, fruits, grains? Great, these are all sources of fiber.

Now, get more specific and write down the actual foods. There is a handout in the appendix to help you with this. I usually recommend that people track their fiber for a few days and get an idea of where they are. Next, gradually work up to 30 grams of fiber a day. I like the number 30 because it can break down evenly between 3 meals and it's enough to make a positive impact on your blood sugar. Ideally, men should ultimately shoot for 38+ grams per day and women 25+ grams. If you choose to eat between meals the extra fiber is even better.

By incorporating a good fiber source at each meal and snack, you can help prevent sharp spikes in blood sugar and insulin levels, which can ultimately help you control your diabetes. As an added bonus, eating a diet that's rich in fiber can also promote healthy gut bacteria, weight loss and help relieve constipation. All good things, right?

Below is a short list of high-fiber plant foods to get you started.

Raspberries: 1 cup = 8 grams

Avocado: 1 cup sliced = 10 grams

Oats: 1 cup cooked = 4 grams

Artichokes: 1 medium = 12 grams

Lentils: 1 cup cooked = 12 grams

Black Beans: 1 cup cooked = 15 grams

Split Peas: 1 cup cooked = 16 grams

Popcorn: 4 cups popped = 5 grams

Almonds: 1 oz = 4 grams

Chia Seeds: 1 oz = 10 grams

Step 3: Choose how you will get your protein.

Be very specific about what you will eat. Will you eat meat or will you choose plant-based protein? Maybe a mixture of both.

Tofu, beans, fish, eggs, milk, yogurt, beef, chicken, pork, wild game? Are there any protein products that don't agree with you? If so, make a note. By "not agree" I mean foods that cause diarrhea, constipation, stomach upset, or any other side effects.

Step 4: Select your healthy fats.

Be specific. Will you focus on nuts, seeds, avocados, olive oil/olives, fish?

Step 5. Review your list.

Your eating style should now stand out quite clearly. By writing down your choices, you have determined what style of eating suits you. Is there anything missing that you really enjoy? If so, write that down as well. Does that food align with your health goals? If not, find ways to work it in occasionally but it may no longer be an "every day" or "every week" food. Consider finding ways to improve the quality of the "less healthy" foods you love so you can enjoy it more often. Get creative.

Now you have your "base food list". Read on as we continue to tweak and individualize your plan so you know exactly what your eating style is.

What is the plan to reverse type 2 diabetes through diet?

The plan is to follow your plan. Follow your own preferred eating style, choosing healthful foods from your list. The base of your eating style is always the non-starchy vegetables, regardless of what eating style you adopt. Focus every day on how you will get enough fiber and non-starchy vegetables to promote fullness and decrease inflammation. Start slowly and incorporate these foods into your diet as you tolerate them.

Start by eating only at mealtimes which means no snacking on the first few days. This will give your body time to start talking to you and letting you know when you actually feel hungry. If you start having physical signs of hunger between meals, then choose a small, basic snack to get you by until your next meal. Ideally, this snack consists of fruits or vegetables and some fat (nuts/seeds).

Let others hop from fad diet to fad diet. Your job is to stick to your preferred eating style (after all, it's what you prefer!) and keep track of your blood sugar. If you consistently get your energy from lean proteins and fats and keep comfortably full with non-starchy veggies and fiber, you should notice a gradual improvement in your numbers.

The best part of eating in an individualized way is that you never feel like you're "cheating." Eating a certain food shouldn't make you feel guilty. This also gives you the flexibility when traveling or attending social events. Your rules give you freedom and flexibility, not rigid structure that constantly leaves you feeling like you've failed.

I'll go into more detail about all the different eating styles later on, but these concepts should hold you over for now (like a little snack).

So when it comes to eating, you are either choosing foods that decrease inflammation or increase it. Food is the root of optimal health and can also be the root of disease. Your gut is the foundation of your whole body's health because over 80% of your immune system is located there. Without a healthy gut, you can't have a healthy immune system. Without a healthy immune system, you're open to infections, inflammation, and disease.

Leaky gut is a term that is not yet fully accepted by all in the medical field but there are years of clinical studies that address it. Leaky gut is also known as intestinal permeability. It is when the tight junctions that hold your intestinal wall together become loose. When that happens, it allows things inside the intestinal tract to permeate to the rest of the body.

Dysbiosis, leaky gut, and inflammation are the root causes of all disease, including diabetes. Any one of those three conditions can trigger the other two. Typically if you have one, you have them all.

Two key genetic tests that can influence your food choices are the Haptoglobin (Hp) variant and Apolipoprotein E genotype (ApoE).

Haptoglobin

When a person with the HP 2-2 genetic variant eats gluten, it produces a by-product called zonulin which is highly inflammatory and loosens the tight junctions in the intestinal lining. A person with this variant cannot clear zonulin from the body in an efficient way. If a person with diabetes has the Hp2-2 variant, they have 5 times the increased risk of cardiovascular disease as compared to Hp1-1 and three times the increased risk compared to Hp2-1. Being a carrier of the Hp2-2 gene in diabetes, compared to carrying an Hp1-1 genotype, can increase the risk of microvascular complications (kidney and eye disease). Studies show that taking 400 IU of vitamin E daily counteracts this increased risk in people with diabetes. Vitamin E is not meant for everyone and can do more harm than good by increasing heart attack risk in some. Don't take it unless you have spoken with your provider.

Apolipoprotein E

The ApoE gene has 3 variants or alleles resulting in 6 genotypes, we each have two alleles, one from each parent.

GENOTYPE	BEST EATING STYLE	% OF POPULATION WITH THIS GENOTYPE
Apo E 2-2, 2-3	Paleo, can tolerate Ketogenic	11% - they have the lowest risk for heart disease. They benefit from a diet with 30-35% of heart healthy fats.
Apo E 3-3, 2-4	Mediterranean	64% - they do better with more plant based foods, healthy fats; typically their best fat content is 25-30% of their diet.
Apo E 3-4, 4-4	Vegetarian, will likely not tolerate ketogenic diet well	25% - they are at highest risk for heart disease. They do best eating <20% of their calories from fat, mostly plant based food, and should limit or avoid alcohol.

This is just one of hundreds of examples of how the food we choose regularly can cause inflammation, depending on our specific genetic makeup. I am not saying that everyone needs to run out and get genetic testing done, but there is new evidence pointing to the benefits of understanding our genetics when it comes to food and treatment for certain disease states.

Having the Apolipoprotein E (ApoE) and Haptoglobin (Hp) genotypes tested can give you some valuable information in regards to individualizing your food choices.

This is also the perfect example of how one element, such as gluten, may cause harm in one person but not in others. A genetic predisposition that increases inflammation in the body could trigger other issues, and ultimately leading to disease. There is a great book called "Beat the Heart Attack Gene" by Dr. Bale and Dr. Doneen. You can take a deeper dive into your heart health as it relates to diabetes and genetics.

We have now reinforced:

1. that diets don't work;
2. that you need a strong "why" to make lasting changes; and
3. how inflammation occurs and affects health.

Let us now move on to discuss the ways to use food as our medicine to begin the healing process for diabetes.

Although weight loss is not the end-all be-all, it is a side effect of decreasing inflammation. We also know from research that when you lose 10% of your body weight within the first 5 years of being diagnosed with diabetes, you have a much better chance of reversing it. So, if you weigh 200 pounds, losing just 20 pounds in 5 years can help reverse diabetes. Focus on the behaviors that will get you there rather than obsessing over the number on the scale.

Below are the 3 principles that make a difference when it comes to individualizing your diet. In my opinion, these are non-negotiable attributes of eating that promote optimal health. Let's talk about quality, quantity and diversity.

The Quality of Ingredients

Quality Carbohydrates

Let's talk about the devil for a minute — you know what I mean, right? Carbohydrates! I'm obviously being a little facetious here. I don't truly believe carbohydrates are the devil but this is a common message heard by people with diabetes. The good news is you don't have to be wary of carbohydrates but you do need to be a little picky.

Carbohydrates can be appreciated for their fiber content. All vegetables are carbohydrates. Foods that grow from the ground or that you pick from the trees are typically carbohydrates. The exceptions are milk and yogurt which have a naturally occurring sugar in them called lactose and are thus categorized as carbohydrates when it comes to diabetes. When you eat carbohydrates closest to their natural form, they tend to contain more fiber. Fiber helps provide the body with energy that lasts longer and also helps keep digestion and blood sugar running smoothly. The process of sprouting grains and soaking legumes will increase the amount of healthy nutrients the body can absorb. Making sure meals are diverse and refraining from large amounts of a single food at one meal can help to balance out nutrient absorption, if there is no time for sprouting and soaking.

Fiber is a very important quality of carbohydrates. Why fiber? It's beneficial in helping with natural weight loss and stabilizing blood sugar, which leads to more energy, less constipation, and improved gut bacteria. Happy bacteria, happy body.

Many of our fiber sources (or carbohydrates) can be exposed to pesticides. Ingesting pesticides can contribute to inflammation. It is important to know where your food comes from and to try to purchase food with minimal contamination. Washing fruits and vegetables helps as does buying organic and locally when possible. This is not a ploy to fill you with fear. The intent is to give you information to make educated decisions about what you put in your body. Our goal is to live a life of optimal health. We want to minimize inflammation as much as possible and what you put in your body (as well as the products you put on your body) absolutely makes a difference. Quality is important — so how do you know if you're eating quality food? You can bet that a food chosen from the produce section, organic or not, is going to be higher in quality than most of the choices you find in the aisles.

Your health depends dramatically on the food choices you make at the store. In general, Americans are not even getting close to the recommended servings of fruits and vegetables per day. I'm not as much concerned about whether your fruits and vegetables are conventional or organic as I am about adding them to your meals every day to begin the reversal of diabetes and heart disease. This is a very important step in achieving optimal health. I've provided further information on carbohydrates as a helpful reference in the carbohydrate guide in the appendix.

Bottomline:

Because we all live in different places and have access to different foods, there is something you must always remember — do the best you can with what you have wherever you are. I live in Alaska and many of my clients who live in remote villages have very limited access to fresh fruits and vegetables, let alone organic items. Many spend hours a day picking berries to freeze to make sure they have enough to last them the winter. Some only have access to frozen or canned vegetables. Do the best you can. If organic foods aren't an option for you, remember it's better to eat conventional fruits and vegetables than none at all. The most important point here is to eat foods as close to nature as possible and, if you have the opportunity to grow, fish, hunt, or pick your own food, that's even better.

Quality Protein

When choosing your source of protein, you can choose animal protein, vegetable protein, or a mixture of both. High quality animal protein comes from wild game, animals that have been grass-fed, wild-caught, treated humanely, organic, and free-range. Because you are eating something that once roamed the land or swam in the seas, you need to consider what the animal ate as well. If you eat wild moose in Alaska, you are likely safe. Animals that live in the wilderness and find their own food will be a high-quality meat source. Animals that are fed food grown with pesticides and given antibiotics won't provide the best quality. It's best to avoid the latter if you can, but the bottom line is to do your best with what is available.

A note about vegetable protein: don't be fooled by the word "vegetarian." Just because that word is on a box doesn't necessarily mean it's healthy. Many frozen, boxed veggie meat products have a lot of ingredients in them that would not be considered high quality.

When choosing a high-quality protein, ask these questions to start: Where did it come from? What did it eat? Was anything added to it?

Quality Fats

When it comes to the quality of fats, you first want to make sure that the type of fat you choose is going to benefit your body and then look at how the fat was processed. Don't be afraid of fat in your food. Choose nuts, seeds, nut butters, avocados, and olives. You will find that eating out poses some challenges when trying to stick to healthy fat options. Salad dressings and oils tend to be lower quality than what you would make at home. Note, even if you are ordering vegetables and fish, you tend to get more than what you paid for and not in a good way. It's still worth choosing the healthiest food possible when eating out. The USDA reports the average American eats foods away from home approximately 4-5 times per week, depending on their socioeconomic status and age. The more meals eat away from home, the less control we have over the quality of food, particularly fats.

The best oils are the one that are high in omega 3's, monounsaturated, and unrefined. Your main cooking oil is ideally olive oil. It has so many health benefits for diabetes and the heart.

For cooking at higher temperatures, try unrefined avocado oil, pay attention to sourcing and reputation of the company you are buying from. If you like the flavor of coconut oil and want to use it occasionally for cooking and baking, choose virgin and unrefined. Coconut oil has lauric acid which is a beneficial component for health.

For salads, flax, safflower and hazelnut are all great for dressings as they are more temperature sensitive. These oils are best stored in the refrigerator.

I highly recommend you check out Lisa Leake's website "100 Days of Real Food" (100DaysofRealFood.com). It's a great starting point, regardless of what eating style you've chosen. There are family-friendly recipes, tips on how to eliminate overly processed food, and how to cook your favorite meals at home.

Quantity

The amount of food that your body needs is relative to your body. This is not information you can acquire from a book. A good place to start is with mindfulness, which means first identifying whether you are actually hungry. The feeling of hunger and the feeling of fullness is the body's built-in way to let you know when you need food and when you've had enough. If you are constantly relying on other people's timelines, work schedules or environmental factors (like time of day, the smell of food or seeing food) to tell you when to eat, then you are likely not getting the proper quantity for your body. Learning to trust your innate ability to respond to hunger and fullness is challenging for many. We've spent a lot of our life ignoring it.

For example, you eat when it's a certain time at school or work. Those specific times might coincide with our natural hunger, but surely not always. Another example is using food as a reward. Eating as a reward for doing something positive throws off our internal measuring system and teaches us to link emotions with food. A final example is eating at events. Enjoying hot dogs and nachos at a ball game or popcorn at the movies is not necessarily "wrong" but, if we are constantly fueling our body when we don't require it, we will start to store the excess. Excess stored fuel is what starts us on the path to disease. The right amount of food for you is determined by listening to what your body tells you.

Many people will tell me that they eat when they don't feel hungry; they just eat because it's time. If this is true for you, then I would challenge you to stop eating by 5–6pm on a given day and then wait and see when you get hungry the next day. This is an experiment to allow your body to actually feel hunger so you can have the opportunity to respond. We will do a deeper dive into mindful eating later on in the book.

Diversity

Diversity in eating is very important for a number of reasons. Diversity helps to keep food interesting to the taste buds. It may also help prevent food sensitivities (a food sensitivity is not the same as an allergy).

When thinking about diversity you want to focus first on

vegetables. Choose vegetables that taste good and try some new ones. Consider eating what is in season. Diversity in vegetables is important to ensure your body functions properly each day. There is no need for "detox" diets when you are eating your vegetables. Vegetables are designed to help the body naturally get rid of what we don't need and build a healthy gut to absorb the precious vitamins and nutrients in our food that we need to function optimally. Choose vegetables that taste good and make you feel good.

Fruit is a hot topic in diabetes. I wanted to discuss it separately from vegetables, although they are often lumped together. Fruit is good for people with diabetes, contrary to popular belief. People with diabetes tend to respond better to lower glycemic fruits such as berries, but if you want to eat mangoes, bananas, grapes, etc., go for it. Just keep quality, quantity and diversity in mind. Advice to avoid fruit needs to be put into context. Drinking fruit juice every day or putting several fruits in a blender and making smoothies may not be the best idea for some people with diabetes. Using fruit as a good source of fiber and sweetness, when needed, is a great plan.

The key here is to pay attention to how much you eat and check your blood sugar to see when enough is enough. If you find certain foods send your blood sugar to the moon, even after you have altered the amount, then you have a choice — eat those foods only occasionally and try to do so on the days you are more active or, if you don't enjoy how they make you feel, you can choose to eliminate them. Ultimately, this is your choice, but it's important to make informed decisions.

For instance, many clients have told me numerous times that bananas are bad for their diabetes yet they choose to eat a high sugar dessert each evening. It's important to understand how foods actually affect your diabetes and to plan a way to enjoy them responsibly. Think about the big picture instead of restricting individual foods.

I've also heard, "I really can't eat bananas, they make my blood sugar go too high. I put them in my cereal yesterday and my blood sugar was 200mg/dl after I ate."

In that scenario, bananas were singled out because they already get a bad rap when it comes to diabetes. Realistically, eating the cereal, milk and banana — all of which are carbohydrates — at the same time can cause blood sugar to go up. It's not just the banana. All carbohydrates are not created equal and, even though all carbohydrates turn to sugar, different people see different results.

If you include grains and beans in your eating pattern, they should be diversified as well. Grains and beans can be tricky. While whole grains and beans are good sources of fiber, some of the proteins in grains can be problematic and some people struggle to process and break them down. Be observant of how your body and your blood sugar respond to the food that you eat. Don't jump to conclusions — particularly if you've eaten a diversified meal. You may have to do some single food experiments.

Sweet tip :

Feel like you don't know how to cook or meal plan? "Living Plate" is my favorite website for helping people brush up on their culinary skills, as well as getting ready-made meal plans created by dietitians. The meal plans are not necessarily created to tell you "how much" to eat, but to spark ideas and help you try new things that you might not otherwise. Check out the resources section in the back of the book for more details.

Bottomline:

Don't eat the same food everyday because you think certain things are "safe." And don't be too quick to add foods to your "never" list. Really test them first. Enjoy life, be creative, keep your taste buds entertained. Variety is the spice of life. When you are able to incorporate more variety, you will feel less restricted and find new foods to love. Your enjoyment of eating will increase and you will finally start to feel satisfied when your body tells you it is full.

CHAPTER 6

Controversies: Should I Avoid Gluten and Fasting Vs Mindful Eating

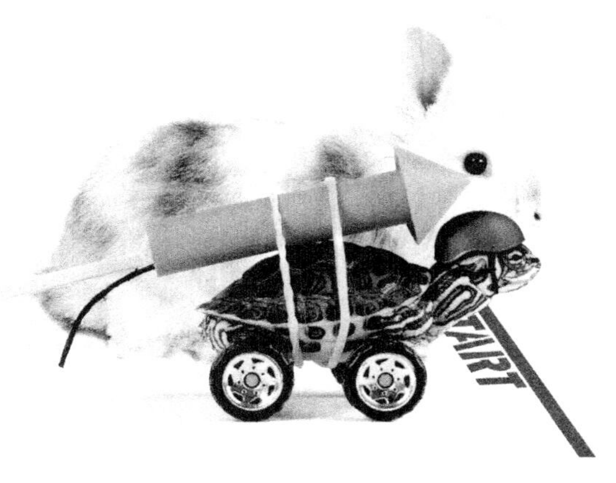

To eat or not to eat gluten — that is the question.

Gluten is a protein in wheat, barley and rye. It's found in a lot of packaged foods, ingredients, and even places you wouldn't expect like cosmetics and pet food. People with celiac disease need to avoid gluten at all costs, but there is also a large portion of the population who have non-celiac gluten sensitivity. Gluten is linked to more than 50 different disease states.

People with autoimmune diseases should strongly consider avoiding gluten and here is why:

In celiac disease (an autoimmune disease), gluten triggers your body to attack cells in your small intestine which damages your microvilli, the barrier of your small intestine. Without microvilli, you can't absorb nutrients properly, which can snowball into a breakdown throughout the body from lack of nutrients. 1 in 133 Americans has celiac disease.

With Hashimoto's disease (autoimmune thyroid disease), consuming gluten can cause the body to become confused and attack thyroid tissue.

Several reports have linked gliadin to type 1 diabetes autoimmunity. Gliadin is one of the proteins in gluten that is responsible for the release of zonulin. Zonulin is a protein that is made in gut and liver cells that can break down the tight junctions of your gut lining, making it "leaky." It is preferable that our gut is not permeable (leaky). Food, waste, bacteria, or any foreign substances in the gut that start leaking out into our bloodstream can often cause inflammation and launch an autoimmune response/attack and ultimately lead to disease.

When a person who has (or is on the verge of) an autoimmune disease eats gluten, it can strengthen the body's attack against its own cells. This is called molecular mimicry and it occurs in many autoimmune conditions. Type 1 diabetes is an autoimmune disease (type 2 diabetes is not) and it can stem from inflammation.

Other diseases associated with gluten (but not limited to): Ankylosing spondylitis, Crohn's disease, rheumatoid arthritis, lupus, type 1 diabetes, multiple sclerosis, schizophrenia, chronic inflammatory demyelinating polyneuropathy and glaucoma (which is believed to have an autoimmune component), neurological disease, autism, chronic fatigue and cancer (brain, breast, lung, ovarian, and pancreatic).

Bottomline:

In some people, gluten can cause the body to attack its own cells if you have an autoimmune disease like one of those described above or if you have non-celiac gluten sensitivity.

I realize the focus here is not autoimmune disease as it pertains to type 1 diabetes, but many people with type 2 diabetes may have some of these other conditions. If that is the case, this section is going to be a very important part of individualizing your eating plan.

One of the key researchers to follow if you are interested in learning more about gluten and the effects it has on the body is Dr. Alessio Fasano. He is Chief of Pediatric Gastroenterology and Nutrition at Mass General Hospital for Children. He directs the Center for Celiac Research, specializing in the treatment of patients of all ages with gluten-related disorders, including celiac disease, wheat allergy, and gluten sensitivity. He conducted a study in 2003 that showed us the actual rate of celiac disease in Americans (1 in 133). If you are looking to read more about the effects of gluten on the body in terms of autoimmune disease, he's a resource I highly recommend.

So who should really avoid gluten?

Let's take this a step further. Think about this for a moment — let's pick a food item you eat all the time (pick a food, any food). If your gut is leaking particles into your bloodstream and your immune system is already "on guard," your body may start to perceive that food as an invader. In reality, it is. That favorite food is supposed to be in your gut, not floating around in your blood. If your immune system starts identifying that food as an invader, you may start having food sensitivity symptoms every time you eat it.

Technically, you could say the root of the problem here is gluten. If gluten wasn't present and triggering zonulin to open the junctions in the gut walls to let anything and everything into the blood, the body's immune system wouldn't be getting all worked up over your beloved food. The good news in this situation is that it's not actually a food "allergy" It's just a sensitivity. Once the leaky gut issue is resolved and the inflammation has calmed, there's a good chance that over time the sensitivity will as well.

Bottomline:

By eating gluten-free foods, you can allow your body to start healing your "leaky gut." That will then keep food and other particles where they are supposed to be and will cut down on food sensitivities.

Still skeptical?

Maybe you're still a little skeptical about this gluten-free business. You should be. This is a big change for you, your family, and your entire eating experience. Here's what you need to know. The gluten of today isn't the same as the gluten of old. Over the years, new strains of wheat have been developed to create fluffier baked goods. These new proteins are foreign to our bodies. They are coming at us in much larger doses than ever before and the body doesn't know how to respond. Gluten is put through a chemical process so it not only makes bread fluffy, but it's now a preservative in your soy sauce or a thickener in your salad dressing. The term "Natural Flavors" is another example of a sneaky place where gluten hides. It's even in personal care products (shampoo, toothpaste, lotions, etc.).

The new strains of wheat that have been created and the abundance of gluten we come in contact with daily have really placed a burden on our immune systems and our bodies are struggling to adapt. Remember, grandma probably wasn't eating a whole lot of packaged food back in the day and was baking her own bread from "older" strains of wheat that had been around for a long time.

How do you know if you have a leaky gut and need to cool it on the gluten? You likely have leaky gut if you already have an autoimmune disease, or experience:

- brain fog, anxiety, depression, joint pain, muscle pain, headaches
- frequently get colds/flu and other infections
- consistent gut issues: diarrhea, bloating, constipation
- gut infections: parasites, bacteria, or fungal overgrowth
- skin issues: eczema, acne, rosacea, psoriasis
- food sensitivities

If you suspect that you may have intestinal permeability (aka leaky gut), reach out to an integrative functional medicine/ nutrition practitioner. Naturopathic doctors, integrative functional registered dietitians, and functional medicine medical doctors are a good place to start.

Some of the top culprits causing leaky gut are:

- gut imbalance related to food intake
- stress
- mold/heavy metals
- surgeries
- foodborne illness
- chemotherapy

- alcohol
- medications such as acid blockers, birth control, NSAIDs, and prednisone

Note: Do not stop any medications without first discussing it with your doctor.

Is gluten-free the miracle cure?

Even though being 100% gluten-free can be very beneficial to some, there is a learning curve. And, yes, it can feel like a miracle cure ... to some. With that said, we also need to look at the downside of gluten-free on your health. Gluten-free can also mean you are eating food that is not as nutrient-dense and has less fiber unless you are really paying attention.

Just one slice of gluten-free bread contains the same amount of energy (or calories) as two slices of regular bread and sometimes little to no fiber. Eating whole wheat (full of gluten) can be a great source of fiber in the diet. As people adopt a gluten-free lifestyle, it's important to choose high-quality products and pay attention to the ingredients. Just because it's gluten-free doesn't mean it's healthy.

Extra non-starchy vegetables are necessary to make up for the fiber/prebiotics that feed our good gut bacteria. Breads and cereals containing gluten were often fortified with extra vitamins and nutrients such as thiamin, folate, iron, and zinc. It's important to ensure you get these nutrients elsewhere if you remove the wheat-based breads, cereals, and pastas.

If you are following a gluten-free diet by choice or due to a medical condition, seek guidance from a dietitian trained in gluten-free diets to make sure you are not consuming any hidden sources of gluten and to make sure your diet is balanced and supporting your good gut bacteria (some prebiotics may be necessary).

A gluten-free diet can be a complete game changer for many people who have autoimmune diseases or gluten sensitivity. Your gut bacteria can make or break your overall health, so be sure to take good care of them whether you are gluten-free or not.

Now that you have taken time to think about your eating style and food preferences, I want to break down some of the more popular eating styles for diabetes. You hear about these "diets" all the time and, for your sanity, it will help to understand them better. In the chart, I've summarized the basics of the eating style, pros and cons, as well as who would benefit from that eating style. Remember, you do not have to follow any of these, but you will see how similar they actually are.

EATING STYLES	**Vegetarian**	**Paleolithic Diet** (traditional). There are many adapted versions of this diet.
BASIC COMPONENTS	Base diet includes vegetables, fruits, grains, beans, seeds, nuts. Occasionally dairy or fish may be eaten, but it depends on the person.	Whole, nutrient-dense foods such as fruit and vegetables, organic meats, eggs, and wild-caught fish. No grains, legumes, dairy, or processed foods.
PROS	Can be healthful if quality, quantity, and diversity are present. High in fiber, which is why it's so beneficial for people with diabetes. Excellent source of magnesium.	This diet is low in sugar, high in vitamins and nutrients, from which many people with diabetes benefit. Many of the higher carbohydrate foods have been removed so there may be a natural lowering of blood sugar.
CONS	Even on a vegetarian diet, people often forget about fruits and vegetables. Instead, their diet is filled with overly processed, packaged foods. This diet is usually low in vitamin D and can be low in iron. Usually need a B12 supplement if it is strictly vegan.	This can be overly restrictive for some. Also, by cutting out grains and legumes, this takes away a large chunk of fiber. So you have to be prudent about eating a lot of vegetables and fruit to keep your fiber intake up.
WHO BENEFITS?	People who need to lower their LDL cholesterol, this is a good eating style. People who don't like meat/fish, regardless of the reason. People who benefit are those who do not have an autoimmune disease. Good for people with APOE 3/4 and 4/4 genotype would benefit from low fat, high carbohydrate style of eating (this is about 25% of people).	Great for people with autoimmune diseases (avoiding nightshades is sometimes an additional recommendation), who prefer low-carb eating, or who need to be gluten-free.

Ketogenic Diet (Keto)	**Mediterranean**
A very low-carb (~20-50 grams a day), high-fat diet. About 70-90% of the diet is made up of fat. This diet has been around for years and originally used in children with epilepsy. Quality is very important; there are many processed foods labeled "keto" that can lead you down the path to deficiencies.	Mostly vegetables, fruits, nuts, legumes, whole grains, herbs, fish/ seafood, extra virgin olive oil. Can have poultry, eggs, cheese and low-fat dairy in moderation. Rare consumption of red meat, anything with added sugar, or overly processed or refined oils. Red wine is allowed in moderation.
Very effective for certain disease states and can be life-altering. Many positive health benefits.	Very inclusive for the most part, not eliminating any major food groups. Has the most research on benefits related to heart health and diabetes.
No grains, so you really have to be strategic in your food choices to make sure your diet is full of fiber and you get the right balance of vitamins and nutrients. Can be challenging to sustain if you don't have a strong motivation or "why" to eat this way. Organ meat is highly recommended in this diet, but for some, this is a little tough to swallow (pun intended). Also, this diet is loaded with vegetables. It's not a bacon and cheese free-for- all as many think.	Depending on where you live, you may not have access to some of these foods or they may not coincide with the food normally consumed in your culture (this could be said for any of these eating styles).
Great for people who have debilitating autoimmune diseases, brain trauma, or just prefer this style of eating. This style of eating may not be ideal for those with liver issues, pancreatic disease, thyroid problems, eating disorders, or gall bladder issues. Often, time restricted feeding or intermittent fasting is combined with this eating style. Typically tolerated better by APOE2/2 or 2/3 genotype.	Anyone. If you are looking for a reasonable eating style for the entire family, this might be a good place to start. It's particularly helpful with lowering triglycerides (as high triglycerides can triple your heart attack risk). Good for people with APOE 2/4 or 3/3 genotypes (this accounts for about 60% of people).

The similarities between all of these is that they all focus on whole, real food, with an emphasis on limiting processed sugar and processed fats/oils. All of these eating styles are great at helping to reverse diabetes. The paleo and keto style of eating is best for people with diabetes who have an underlying autoimmune disease.

As you read about the different eating styles, did one style appeal more to you than the other? Which one looked the easiest? There's nothing wrong with hitting the easy button.

Bottomline:

There is evidence to support each eating style. There are many healthcare professionals who feel strongly about one or the other. The problem lies in trying to translate a clinical study into real life for the general population. Culture, accessibility, cost, and food preferences all need to be addressed and one style of eating does not serve everyone. Don't get me wrong, many people are successful at picking a diet, sticking to it long-term and seeing great results. But if you're not one of those people (I'm not either), let's forge ahead and see what eating style appeals to you so that you have a general roadmap for eating to reverse diabetes. You already made your list of preferred foods a few chapters back.

Which one lined up most closely to the list you made? Did you learn anything new about why one eating style might be a better fit for you?

The best part is you don't have to follow any of these exclusively. The key takeaway and the basis of most of these eating styles are the non-starchy vegetables, high fiber, low glycemic fruits, healthy fats, and quality proteins. The only thing that really varies is the percentage of the macronutrients (fats, proteins, carbohydrates). Not every eating style works for every person. Identifying with an eating style doesn't mean you can never alter it or choose a food that doesn't fall within its structure. It just gives you more clarity. Once you have a style in mind, meal planning and preparation become easier.

Fiber and Carbohydrates

The hardest decision often comes with the carbohydrate group. Carbohydrates are responsible for raising blood sugar, so finding the type and amount that you can handle is worth exploring. Some people do not break down starchy carbohydrates very well (grains, beans, legumes) and it can cause a lot of GI upset, inflammation and, as we learned earlier, some people are sensitive to gluten.

So pay attention to how food makes you feel. If you are unsure about a food, remove it for at least 4 weeks, then add it back and note any changes. Most Americans do not get enough fiber, so that may be part of the problem as well. Gradually increase your fiber over time. If you still have gut issues, you may need to single out certain foods.

People with diabetes benefit from fiber and resistant starch (nuts, seeds, legumes, unripe bananas, cooled rice/pasta). Eating a lot of fruits, vegetables, nuts and seeds which are high in fiber can increase butyrate production. Butyrate is a short chained fatty acid (SCFA) that has been linked to improved blood sugar by increasing the body's GLP1 production and improving insulin sensitivity. This is more evidence that feeding your gut bacteria what it needs to flourish is an essential part of managing blood sugar. On the flip side, some food choices can damage the gut bacteria.

Sugar Cravings

One of the most common topics clients talk about are sugar cravings. I think most will agree that eating excess amounts of sugar is a problem. Some people rely on quick, processed foods, especially for snacks or dealing with emotions. Since these products often contain added sugar, it makes up a large proportion of their daily calorie intake. The Center for Disease Control (CDC) reported in 2005–2010 that the average percentage of total daily calories in adults from added sugars was 13%. In 2020, they recommended this be decreased to 10%. The goal is to keep added sugar intake to less than 13 teaspoons or less per day, yet most Americans get more than 3 times this amount. High sugar intake has been linked to many medical conditions such as heart disease, diabetes, obesity, and some types of cancer. Sugar has addictive properties: the more you eat, the more you crave. This is why after certain holidays that are heavy on the sweets, it can feel harder to kick the habit.

When we eat sugar, endorphins and serotonin are released in the body. These hormones help to regulate our mood and help us feel happy. Some people eat sugary foods for emotional reasons and for others, it's a habit. They are used to eating something sweet after a meal. People who have diabetes may crave sugar when their blood sugar levels drop too low or go really high. When blood sugar is low, people feel hungry, angry, and often crave sweets. In this case, sugar is beneficial - especially if they take insulin or a medication that can cause low blood sugar. If someone's blood sugar is too high, this can also cause sugar cravings. When blood sugar is high, the sugar is not in the cells where it needs to be for the body to use it as energy. When the cells do not have access to the sugar, they send the message that more sugar is needed which can lead to sugar cravings.

Calcium, zinc, chromium, and magnesium imbalances can also manifest themselves as sugar cravings. We are not demonizing sugar, but rather looking at the facts. There is an expectation that some of us will choose to have sugar on occasion such as desserts or candy. However, it's important to watch the effects on blood sugar and decide when and how often you should choose to incorporate sweets. Beyond raising blood glucose as previously noted, too much sugar leads to inflammation. Inflammation leads to gut permeability and, eventually, disease. With regard to the good-hearted friends and family members who remind you to go easy on the sugar because you have diabetes, they can benefit from that advice as well.

What about artificial sweeteners?

Within the overarching theme of keeping food close to nature, artificial sweeteners do not fit in well. However, some people have found that using them in place of added sugars has been beneficial for weight loss and cavity prevention. If you choose to use them, do so sparingly just as you would sugar. If you wouldn't drink regular soda daily, then refrain also from drinking diet drinks daily. You could consider stevia leaf extract and monk fruit as alternatives, they are not considered artificial sweeteners. Some will also use sugar alcohols, also known as polyols (sorbitol, xylitol, mannitol,maltitol, etc), which only have half the effect on blood sugar as regular sugar. Sugar alcohols are typically found in products labeled "sugar free" or "no sugar added." Careful with sugar alcohols, because if you overdo it, they can cause bloating and diarrhea.

Evidence on the long-term safety of artificial sweeteners is mixed and they may disrupt the balance of your friendly gut bacteria. By now I'm sure you have a good idea of how I feel about good gut bacteria - preserve and protect is the name of the game! Better safe than sorry.

Bottomline:

Even with sugar substitutes, quantity still matters.

Your body adapts.

Many people are living with diabetes for years before they know they have it. Sometimes their blood sugar can climb quite high. Normal blood sugar is 70-120 mg/dl. Over time, if blood sugar climbs higher and higher, the body adapts. The person may feel more tired but they write it off to aging or being really busy. A person can walk around and be "functioning" with blood sugar in the 200-300mg/dl range and not know it. Eventually when diabetes is diagnosed and measures are taken to lower their blood sugar, they become more sensitive to the highs. Some will say they feel hot, tired, or run down when their blood sugar rises and they can feel it. They didn't necessarily have that feeling before because the 200-300 range was their norm and their body adapted.

My point here is that the body is constantly adapting. If you take in a high amount of sugar and try to stop, you will probably miss it and you may feel that nothing tastes sweet enough. But, if you gradually lower your intake over time, your body will adapt. Eventually, if you eat something sweet, it may overwhelm you and you may not be able to tolerate it.

Sweet Tip :

Sugar is highly inflammatory but tastes good to most of us. If you choose to eat it, make sure it's high priority and worthy of a detour from your typical eating. If it's not worthy of your taste buds and it's a bump in blood sugar, ditch it and move on. Also notice in the previous chart that sugar intake was limited among every single eating style. You should definitely savor and enjoy your sweet treats when you choose to have them but doing so should not be a cause for feeling guilty. Guilt is not a welcome companion on our journey to optimal health.

Can I just NOT eat?

Now that's an interesting question to ask! Over the past few years, there's been more and more talk about the possible benefits of fasting. People have been fasting for centuries. Hippocrates and the Greeks must have been on to something. They are responsible for the Mediterranean Diet and found fasting was a beneficial practice for many health conditions. Contrary to the typical advice of eating every few hours, the majority of fasts require 12–24 hours of no energy intake or very low calorie intake. There are many different types of fasting so here's a quick look at all of them and what they are.

TYPE OF FASTING	DEFINITION	POSSIBLE BENEFITS	LEVEL OF DIFFICULTY(IN MY OPINION)
Intermittent fasting (IF)	A fasting day alternated with 1-6 days of normal diet; often consuming 20-25% of total calorie needs on the "fasting" day	Decrease in abdominal fat and blood pressure. Anti-aging.	Moderate
Time-restricted feeding	Eating within specific time windows; common time frames are: 12-13 hour overnight fast or 16 hour fast/8 hour feeding	Improved immune system, increased insulin sensitivity. A 12-week study showed that when people with diabetes ate between the hours of 8 am - 4 pm, they saw a decrease in fatty liver disease and better glucose tolerance.	Easiest
Alternate day fasting	Eating every other day	Decrease body fat and insulin levels	Difficult. Studies show a high drop-out rate

TYPE OF FASTING	DEFINITION	POSSIBLE BENEFITS	LEVEL OF DIFFICULTY(IN MY OPINION)
Prolonged fasting (PF)	Water only for 2 or more consecutive days	May protect against adverse effects of chemotherapy. PF followed by a vegetarian diet can decrease pain and inflammation in people with rheumatoid arthritis	Difficult
Protein restriction	Restriction of certain essential amino acids	Possible protection from chronic diseases, such as cancer; improved insulin sensitivity	Moderate

Who might want to try fasting:

- anyone with the desire to see what it is all about and experience possible health benefits
- anyone willing to commit and follow through for at least a month to give it a solid chance
- anyone interested in improving immune function and insulin sensitivity
- anyone wondering if this might jumpstart weight loss for them

Who should think twice about trying it or discussing it first with their healthcare professional who has researched and understands fasting:

- anyone on insulin or a sulfonylurea (glipizide, glyburide, glimepiride)
- anyone with adrenal fatigue/severe stress for long periods of time
- anyone who has struggled with disordered eating or an eating disorder
- anyone with any other disease or condition that could be worsened by going long periods without eating

If you decide this is for you, the easiest one to start with would be the time-restricted overnight fast for 12–13 hours. Most people do this one as a matter of routine anyway but, if you don't, it might be the easiest one to start with because the majority of the fast happens while you're sleeping.

Fasting is a practice that's been around for a very long time. Even though it appears to be the latest fad, people have been doing this for centuries. There is definitely a right and wrong way to fast so do a little research.

Finally, ask yourself why you want to do it. Your "why" is what drives your will. For example, if you've chosen to do the time-restricted feeding because you heard you can "eat whatever you want" during the 8 hour time-frame, this truly might not be the right choice for you. You are likely to be disappointed in your results and do more harm than good. If your "why" is to improve your sleep and/or your immune system or some other health issue, then you will be more motivated to provide your body with the highest quality food during your eight-hour feeding time to help support your "why."

I encourage taking chances and trying new things that are reasonable. Intermittent fasting (IF) and time-restricted feeding are harmless to most people and could be beneficial. This concept also appears to completely contradict our next topic, so I want to take a moment to explain. Before you ever think about trying fasting, you first need to learn to become a mindful eater to be successful. If you are a hardcore emotional eater and you try fasting, you will fail time and again and likely feel terrible about it. So remember, fasting is a tool you can use but it's important to select the right tool at the right time.

Now let's move on to how to become a mindful eater and why it is one of the most freeing concepts you may ever learn!

Mindful Eating & Diabetes

When it comes to managing your diabetes, what you eat is important (I realize I'm not telling you anything you don't already know - yet). Believe it or not, when and how you eat is just as important. Mindless eating (i.e., eating while doing other things) can impact what and how much you eat. On the flipside, mindful eating (i.e., being attentive and present while you eat) can help you take charge of your diabetes.

Mindless eating can wreak havoc on your health and get in the way of managing your diabetes. Some common mindless eating habits to ditch are:

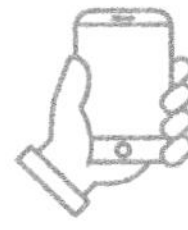

Eating while watching TV or browsing on your phone.

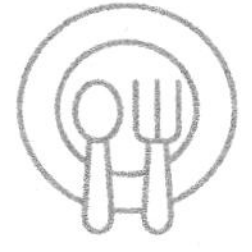

Finishing everything on your plate when you're no longer hungry.

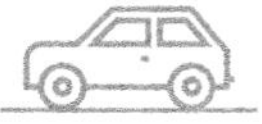

Eating while driving.

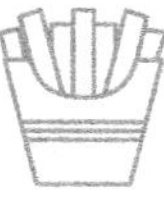

Eating while standing up and/or out of a bag.

Mindful eating is all about being aware of your experiences and noticing your physical hunger and satiety cues. Some popular mindful eating habits are:

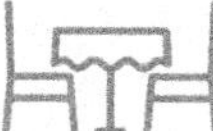

Eating in a designated spot for meals, such as the kitchen table rather than the couch or bed.

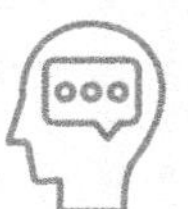

Listening to your body's hunger and fullness cues and responding appropriately.

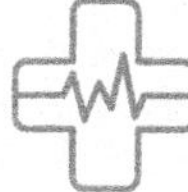

Noticing how you feel after eating certain foods or meals.

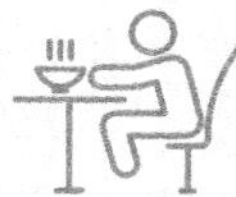

Eating slowly and chewing your food thoroughly.

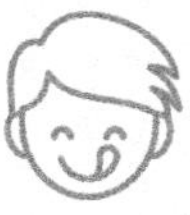

Being present and engaging all of your senses while you eat.

Believe it or not, the incidence of diabetes can be reduced by almost 60% with mindfulness-focused lifestyle interventions. In a pilot study published in the ***Journal of the Academy of Nutrition and Dietetics***, training in mindful eating and diabetes self-management helped to improve food intake, weight loss, and blood sugar control.

In this study, adults with type 2 diabetes were given a mindful eating intervention that was modified for diabetes self-management. In addition to basic nutrition information, they learned about mindful meditation, mindful eating, and awareness of hunger and satiety cues. Three months later, the participants reported weight loss, cognitive control over eating, enhanced self-confidence, decreased overeating, and less eating beyond satiety. These findings demonstrate that training in "mindful eating" can help manage diabetes and encourage healthy eating habits.

Another study found that incorporating mindfulness into a diet-exercise program may promote long-term improvement in metabolic health and obesity. Engaging in mindful eating may contribute to long-term decreases in the eating of sweets and fasting blood glucose levels.

Let's take a moment to reflect on how awesome this is! You don't have to count calories or measure out food. You simply take into account what sounds good to you and what would be most nourishing for your body. You then remove distractions, take a bite, savor it, and when you start to feel full you stop. Sounds simple and amazing, right? We were all born with an innate ability to do this, but situations during our life may have muted this ability. We need to bring it back. Here's how.

SCALE: How Hungry Am I?

TIME TO EAT
I COULD EAT
but could also wait a little if needed
NO FOOD NECESSARY
1 So hungry you could eat a horse
2 Starving
3 Hungry
4 Stomach growling and slight pangs
5 Satisfied - not hungry, not full ... content
6 Full - feel food, but not uncomfortable
7 Really Full
8 Unbutton pants, slight discomfort
9 Stuffed, severe discomfort
10 Sick - could vomit, feel like exploding

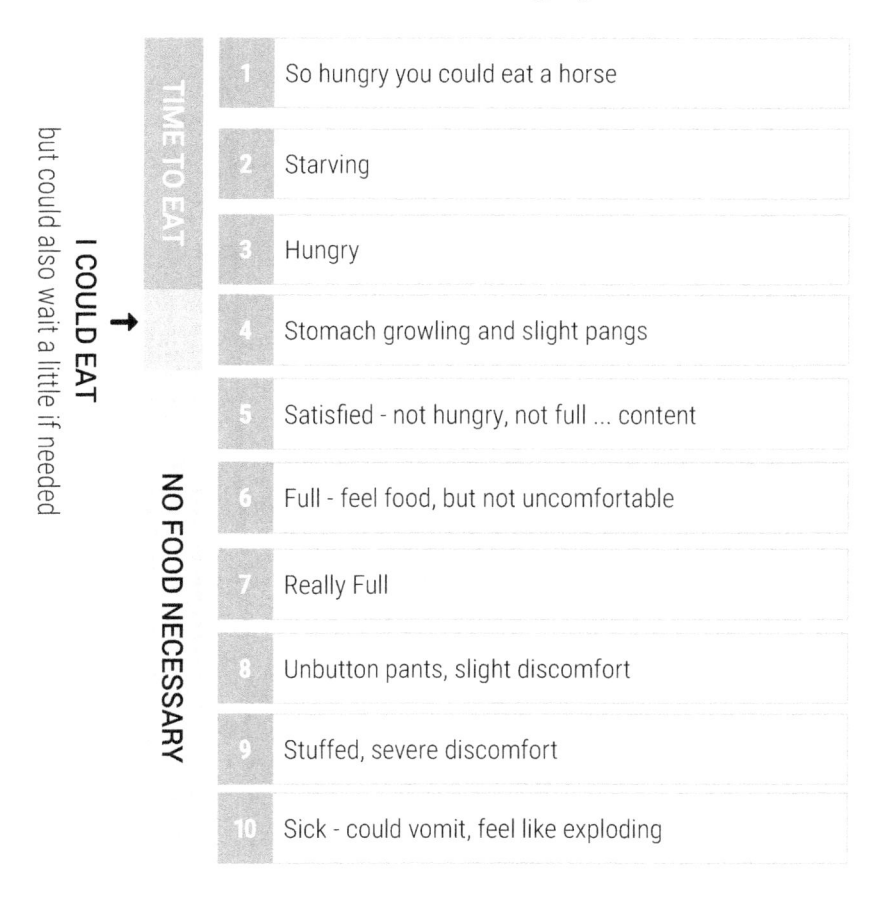

How to Eat Mindfully

Below are four steps you can take to get started with mindful eating. Identify where you are on the above scale prior to eating, then re-evaluate 15 minutes or so after eating. The goal is to vary between a 3 to 6 most of the day. If you notice your ratings frequently fall above or below those numbers, start evaluating what needs to be done differently to get into that target range.

1. Don't wait until you're starving to sit down and have a meal. If you wait to eat until you're ravenous, you'll find yourself eating more food, faster, and not stopping when you're full.

2. Appreciate the eating experience. Take a moment to appreciate and express your gratitude about the food you're eating and who you're eating it with. This can bring a great deal of enjoyment to your table.

3. Chew your food thoroughly and slowly. Taking the time to chew your food thoroughly and slowly is good for digestion and can enhance the enjoyment of food by releasing more flavor.

4. Engage your senses. While you're cooking and eating your food, take note of the flavors, colors, textures, smells, and sounds that are associated with the different foods.

The next meal you eat after reading this would be the perfect time to try it out. Already a mindful eater? See if you can take it to the next level by really slowing down and savoring!

Is there a discrepancy between mindful eating and fasting?

Excellent question! I'm so glad you asked — it means you're paying attention! Yes, there absolutely is a discrepancy and we briefly touched on it earlier. Mindful eating is most important because it's an innate and inherent attribute that can give us lasting results. Deciding whether or not to fast will not make or break you. On the other hand, the act of mindful eating allows you to feed your body on your terms and to recognize exactly what and how much you need. It's also the best way to determine what food your body responds to best. Taking a moment after eating to assess if you feel better or not will give you valuable insight as to what foods fuel you best. Fasting on the other hand is asking you to ignore those feelings of hunger, push through and eat by the clock. You can still utilize mindful eating techniques during the "feeding period" of your fasting practice. Fasting is just a tool and many people will fail at using that tool if they have not mastered the mindful eating part. If you get great results using fasting as a tool in addition to mindful eating, then some form of fasting can become a way of life for you.

The Nutrition of Diabetes

If you've ever been to a diabetes class or visited with a dietitian, you are sure to have come across a food label. We will touch briefly on this because people are often looking at the wrong parts of the label.

When reading a food label, first look at the ingredients underneath the label. The ingredients give you a little more perspective on what you are reading in the nutrition facts. Remember quality, quantity and diversity? If you see a lot of ingredients you don't recognize or find substandard, it's likely a wise idea to forgo this item.

If the ingredients are acceptable to you, move on to the nutrition facts label. Look at the serving size first. Everything on the label is describing what is in one serving. Next, it's up to you. If you are trying to increase your fiber intake, start there. Most of your staple carbohydrate foods should have around 3g fiber per serving, or more.

Note: If you want to keep it simple and save yourself some time, choose lots of fruits and vegetables that don't have labels. Easy, right?

Note: If it's there's a food that you're "craving" and it's not the healthiest choice, you have two options: 1) either don't look at the label, just buy it, eat it and enjoy it; or 2) see if there is a more healthful version of it or if it's something you could make on your own to improve the quality.

Bottomline:

When it's an "occasional" food, just enjoy it. When it's a daily or frequent food, scrutinize the label like a detective. The foods we eat every day send messages to our body. What kind of messages are you sending?

Nutrition Facts

8 servings per container

Serving size **1 cup (68g)**

Amount per serving

Calories **370**

	% Daily Value
Total Fat 5g	**7%**
Saturated Fat 1g	**3%**
Trans Fat 0g	
Cholesterol 0mg	**0%**
Sodium 150mg	**6%**
Total Carbohydrate 48g	**15%**
Dietary Fiber 5g	**14%**
Total Sugars 13g	
Includes 10g Added Sugars	**20%**
Protein 12g	

Vit. D 2mcg 10%	Calcium 210 mg 20%
Zinc 7mg 50%	Biotin 300mg 100%

* The % Daily Value (DV) tells you how much a nutrient in a serving of food contributes to a daily diet. 2,000 calories a day is used for general nutrition advice.

Sugar Information

Sugars are included in the total carbohydrates so don't add them up separately. Also take a look at the ingredients and remember: less is more. The ingredients are listed in order of weight. So if sugar is the first or second ingredient, you know that it makes up a lot of that particular food.

As discussed earlier, dietary guidelines suggest limiting calories from added sugar to less than 10% per day, which for most would be 13 teaspoons or less. Experts believe that sugar consumption is a major cause of obesity and many chronic diseases such as diabetes.

Bottomline:

What you eat is really important when it comes to managing your diabetes. Eating a diet that's full of fruits and vegetables can make your diabetes much more manageable. Processed foods can really take a toll on your blood sugar and energy levels. By choosing whole foods instead, you increase the fiber which can help regulate your blood sugar. By incorporating a good fiber source at each meal and snack, you can help prevent sharp spikes in blood sugar and insulin levels, which can ultimately give you more energy and stabilize blood sugar. No one is asking you to be perfect, you will definitely eat food that is not considered healthy, and life will go on. The focus is to try to keep the base of your diet as healthy as possible, this is what will lead you to optimal health.

CHAPTER 7

How Do I Incorporate These Eating Principles into My Busy Life?

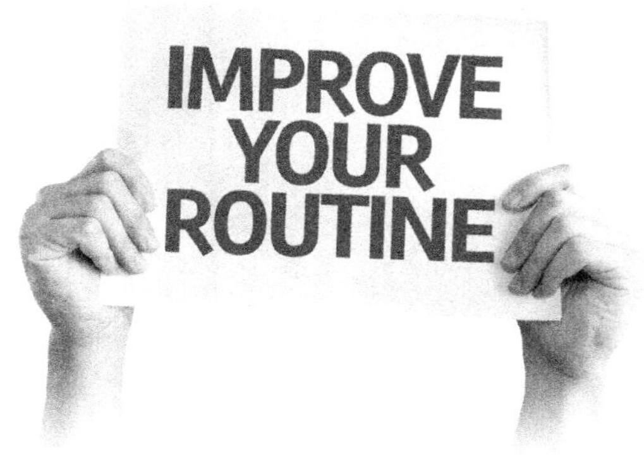

Change starts with a strong "why" and a decision to make it happen. Many people have an all or nothing mindset. They go all in, get overwhelmed and quit. Something to remember during this process is that slow and steady wins the race. It could be that you've been on the right path for a while now. While it's admirable that you want to reverse diabetes and take charge of your health, it doesn't mean all that should happen by tomorrow. Picking one or two small things to change, however, will help give you some immediate results. Now that you have all this information, let's make your individualized plan.

To fast or not to fast, that is the question.

Is This Behavior for Me?

Have I ever been told I have "adrenal fatigue"?
Have I been highly stressed for a very long time?

YES.
Keep your fast to a simple 12-13 hour overnight fast. If you want to try a longer fasting period, work with your healthcare provider closely before transitioning, in case medications need to be adjusted.

NO.
You are a candidate for a longer fasting period.

How to Implement

16-hour fast: 8-hour feed or a modified version. Can try anything from 13- to 16-hour fast and then pick your feeding period and stick with it!

Why am I Doing this?

Helps improve sleep, immune function, insulin resistance, and sometimes weight loss.

Non-negotiable: Non-starchy Vegetables

Is This Behavior for Me?

This one is the KEY to reversing or slowing the progression of diabetes.

YES.

Start by writing down your favorite vegetables that you know you will eat. Then make a list of some you would be willing to try. Ask your friends for their favorite vegetable recipe. Better yet, ask them to make it for you!

NO.

Ha, trick question! No is not an option if you are serious about reversing diabetes. This form of medicine is the most impactful and will make or break your reversal.

How to Implement

Stock the fridge with vegetables. Pick veggies that are easy to grab and require little prep. Buy them already prepped/cut, if needed. Take a cooking class or knife skills class to help you feel more confident in food prep.

Why am I Doing this?

Lower blood sugar, feed good gut bacteria, increase feeling of fullness, and decrease sugar cravings.

Do you have an autoimmune disease or genetic conditions that accompany your type 2 diabetes, such as multiple sclerosis, lupus, Hashimoto's, rheumatoid arthritis? Do you know your genetics regarding Haptoglobin?

Is This Behavior for Me?

Avoiding gluten and dairy can be a good start toward reducing inflammation in chronic disease, especially if you have an accompanying autoimmune disease. If you have the Haptoglobin,1-2 or 2-2 variant, eating gluten can increase your risk of having a heart attack, especially when you have type 2 diabetes. You would need to get a genetic test for this to make a determination.

YES.

If you answered yes, then choose either gluten or dairy to start with. (See list of anti-inflammatory gluten-free foods in appendix.)

NO.

If not, then you can incorporate all food groups. Focus on the highest quality food from each group, in particular, the grains. Choose the highest fiber.

How to Implement

Start with the foods you can eat (see list in appendix). Sticking with whole foods makes it easier because you don't have to review labels.

Why am I Doing this?

To heal leaky gut, to feel better and ultimately increase quality of life.

Non-negotiable:
Exercise

Is This Behavior for Me?

Pay attention to any body parts that need special care such as knees, shoulders, etc. and pick a movement that can help.

YES.

Decide what time of day you have the most energy and would be most likely to exercise.

NO.

Start with a reasonable amount of time that you know you can be successful with. 5 minutes counts!

How to Implement

Decide what type of exercise would work best for me right now?

Why am I Doing this?

Remind yourself that this is your medicine. Taking your medicine daily is important. You can change up how intense your exercise is, or how long, but get in a habit of moving daily.

"A dream is just a dream, but a goal is a dream with a plan and a deadline." **Harvey McKay**

Earlier in the book, we discussed that 95% of the actions we take are subconscious and only 5% are conscious. The best way to help incorporate new principles, therefore, is to do a daily meditation. Daily meditation helps to reprogram our subconscious.

The reason this is necessary and beneficial is that I suspect you want long-lasting change. You are choosing new actions and behaviors that you believe will support the future healthy you. Making sure these changes stick is really important.

Let's break down one of these healthy behaviors and how you could start applying it.

Goal: Add more vegetables and ultimately get up to 6+ cups daily.

Before you go to bed at night, do some deep breathing. Focus on your favorite vegetable dishes, think about the flavors and how good you feel when you eat vegetables. Remind yourself that you are a vegetable lover. When you wake up in the morning, the first thing you do in the kitchen is grab a vegetable, eat a carrot stick or broccoli floret; it doesn't even have to be a whole serving. You are just reminding yourself that you are a vegetable lover. Moving on with your day, consider adding spinach to your eggs or taking extra vegetables to eat with your lunch. By beginning your day eating a vegetable and ending the day thinking about vegetables, you are starting to reprogram how you think. If you are under the notion that you don't like vegetables and, thus, rarely eat them – chances are that won't change. What you think about can become a habit.

What I have just described is the secret to making behavior changes work. If you just rely on willpower, that muscle easily becomes overworked. Program your subconscious mind to adopt these new attitudes and behaviors so they become automatic, just like all those old habits did. It's one thing to know what to do and another thing to actually do it. I can't tell you the number of times I have heard people say "I already know what to do, I just need to do it."

CHAPTER 8

How Does Sleep Affect Diabetes?

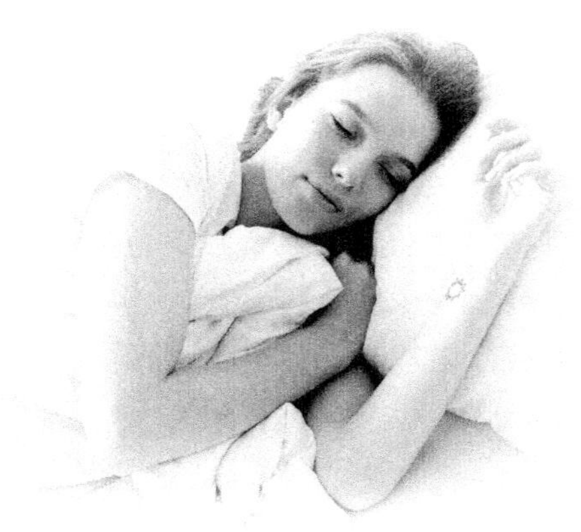

Not getting enough sleep can be detrimental to your health – particularly if you have diabetes. Many assume that while you're sleeping, your brain isn't doing all that much. Believe it or not, it's quite the opposite! Key hormones are regulated while you sleep – insulin, stress hormones, growth hormones, hunger hormones, etc. This is also the time when your body restores, repairs, and strengthens itself and, in particular, your immune system.

Hormones are involved in almost every aspect of our life. Sleep experts have determined that inadequate sleep can change your hormones (and gut bacteria). This ultimately impacts food choices, weight, and blood sugar. Disruption of your circadian rhythm can cause hormonal dysfunction and wreak havoc on your health, causing metabolic diseases like diabetes and obesity.

Diabetes and Sleep

Sleep deprivation is a significant risk factor for type 2 diabetes but it's often overlooked by medical professionals. If you don't get enough sleep on a regular basis, your body will release less insulin after you eat and start producing more stress hormones that will keep you awake. Cortisol is an important hormone when it comes to sleep. It helps wake us up in the morning, maintains our energy throughout the day and, ideally, it drops at night so we can rest. When cortisol remains elevated, it can impact sleep duration and quality.

These stress hormones, like cortisol, actually suppress insulin and increase the release of sugar. Oftentimes people with diabetes, particularly those who are stressed, will see higher blood sugar levels when they wake up, even if they went to bed with their blood sugar within target range.

3 reasons some people wake up with high blood sugar

1. A big dinner that is high in carbohydrates and saturated fat. Saturated fat creates insulin resistance, and slows the release of glucose into the blood leading to higher morning readings.

2. Your liver dumped a little sugar into your blood overnight while insulin levels were low. Then as your "wake up" hormones started getting active around 4AM, they blocked your insulin from working as well and triggered the release of sugar into the blood which leads to higher blood sugar than when you went to bed – aka Dawn Phenomenon.

3. Maybe you use insulin and you had a little too much on board over night, your sugar may have dropped too low and then rebounded from a surge of hormone – this is called the Somogyi Effect. It is a less common occurrence and tends to happen more in people with Type 1 diabetes or those with type 2 diabetes who take insulin. A continuous

glucose monitor can help here or waking up and doing a fingerstick for a couple nights to see if you catch any low blood sugars. Another sign of Somogyi is if you wake up and can tell you were sweating a bit more than usual (for no apparent reason), signaling a possible low blood sugar reaction overnight.

Note: Avoid snacking before bed (too much carbohydrate and not a lot of movement can cause high blood sugars). On the flip side, try a very small snack before you go to sleep (sometimes a little snack can stop your liver from dumping sugar into your blood)... keyword small - something with fat and/or fiber. Certain vitamin deficiencies can create more insulin resistance. Last but not least, exercise is always a winner. Exercise can affect blood sugar for days.

Depending on which research study you read, anywhere from 50–70% of people with diabetes also have sleep apnea. If you snore, wake up with headaches, or your significant other tells you that you stop breathing at times during the night - be sure to talk to your doctor about your risk for sleep apnea. Untreated sleep apnea can increase the risk of high blood pressure, heart problems, depression and obesity, to name a few. Let's dive a little deeper into some of these relationships to sleep.

Obesity and Sleep

Insulin isn't the only hormone impacted by sleep. According to the ***National Sleep Foundation***, two hormones that help regulate hunger (ghrelin and leptin) are impacted by sleep quality and quantity. Ghrelin (our hunger hormone) increases your appetite, while leptin (our satiety hormone) decreases it. When you don't get enough sleep, these important hormones get out of whack.

Ghrelin is a hormone produced in your gastrointestinal tract. It tells your brain that you are hungry. Ghrelin increases when your stomach is empty and decreases when full. Most people feel the affects of ghrelin when they start a new diet, as they immediately feel hungrier after restricting calories. You can naturally lower ghrelin by increasing muscle (lifting weights), avoiding extreme eating (under/overeating), eating protein with each meal, getting plenty of sleep at night, and avoiding drastic weight changes.

Leptin is a hormone that is produced by your body's fat cells. This hormone tells the brain you are satisfied and no further energy is required. But just as cells can become insulin resistant, they can also become leptin resistant. This is a problem because leptin also has several other important functions related to fertility, immunity, fat storage, and the brain.

Fat cells release leptin for two reasons:

1. High levels of leptin tell your brain that you have plenty of fat stored.

2. Low levels tell your brain that fat stores are low and that you need to eat.

It's easy to see how this could be a problem. If a person is overweight and has excess fat cells, they are producing more leptin. Ideally, this should tell the brain that fat is present, to stop requiring energy and to burn energy at a normal rate. With sleep deprivation, that is not what happens. Leptin resistance is one of the main reasons why people who are overweight or obese have a hard time losing weight. Their brain keeps sending signals to eat because it's not getting the memo from leptin that fat stores are plentiful.

A study published in ***European Journal of Clinical Nutrition*** combined the results of 11 studies with a total of 172 participants. Researchers found that partial sleep deprivation resulted in an increased energy intake of 385 calories per day.

Sleep deprivation also impacts your motivation for exercise. Think about it. Do you feel like going to the gym after 4 hours of sleep? Probably not. And even if you make it to the gym, you'll be far more sluggish and less productive than if you got 7–8 hours of sleep.

It is important to recognize this vicious cycle. Excess body weight increases the risk of sleep apnea. Sleep apnea leads to sleep deprivation. Sleep deprivation causes an increase in leptin, where your body craves high-carb foods and salty snacks, which in turn prevents weight loss. And the cycle continues...

Diabetes and Sleep Apnea

Sleep apnea, also known as obstructive sleep apnea (OSA), changes how your body processes sugar, promotes insulin resistance, and is associated with developing type 2 diabetes. People with sleep apnea often have low vitamin D. Having low vitamin D can worsen the negative impact of sleep apnea on heart health. Sleep apnea increases inflammation in the body and oxidative stress (cell damage). While a healthy diet is important in general, it's even more important for someone with sleep apnea.

Vitamins A, C, D, E, in addition to selenium, copper, magnesium, glutathione, copper, and N-acetyl-cysteine all work in the body to shield it from the effects of sleep apnea and to actually help restore and heal the body.

VITAMIN/ NUTRIENT	FOODS TO EAT:
Vitamin A1 - people with sleep apnea often have low retinol levels (A1).	Fatty oily fish, liver, cheese and butter. If you can't eat or don't like some of these foods, you may need to consider a vitamin A1 or retinol supplement. Be careful with dosing; talk to your provider/dietitian first if you are pregnant or considering pregnancy. Don't exceed 25,000 IU/7500 mcg RAE unless being supervised.
Vitamin C	Citrus fruit, berries, bell peppers, chili peppers, pineapple, potatoes, brussels sprouts. Foods high in Vitamin C can improve blood vessel health.
Vitamin D	Fatty oily fish (salmon, sardines, herring, safe- catch tuna), egg yolks, grass-fed red meat, liver, mushrooms, cod liver oil.
Vitamin E	Nuts and seeds. Helps with oxidative stress.
Selenium	Pork, beef, turkey, chicken, fish, shellfish, and eggs. Powerful antioxidant to reduce oxidative stress and possibly help with snoring.
Copper	Liver, organ meats, oysters, lobster, spirulina, shiitake mushrooms, nuts, seeds, leafy greens, dark chocolate. Many people with sleep apnea have low levels of an enzyme that breaks down harmful molecules, called superoxide dismutase (SOD). Copper is a cofactor, meaning you need copper to have SOD.

VITAMIN/ NUTRIENT	FOODS TO EAT:
Magnesium	Green leafy vegetables, nuts, avocado, dark chocolate, potatoes, bananas, black beans. Mg helps with relaxation and regulating your stress response.
Glutathione	Broccoli, Brussels sprouts, cauliflower, kale, watercress, mustard greens, spinach, avocados, asparagus, okra, garlic, shallots, onions, high quality beef, fish, poultry. Studies show the sleep apnea can worsen or cause liver damage (fatty liver disease), and being deficient in certain antioxidants, such as glutathione, can exacerbate this. It also helps reduce the impact of oxidative stress.
N-Acetyl Cysteine (NAC)	Beans, lentils, spinach, bananas, salmon, tuna, chicken, turkey, yogurt, cheese, eggs, sunflower seeds. Helps to restore glutathione, decrease inflammation and oxidative damage. Your body needs adequate folate, B6 and B12 vitamins to produce cysteine.

As you can see from the food list in the chart, a variety of vegetables, colorful fruits, nuts, seeds, whole grains, and high-quality protein can be medicine for sleep apnea.

5 Tips to Improve Your Sleep

Getting consistent sleep is a great way to manage your diabetes and help support your body's ability to regulate its blood sugar. Here are 5 tips to help you improve your sleep.

1. Stick to a sleep routine. This means waking up and going to bed at the same time every single day – including weekends. Consistency is key! This is especially important if you have diabetes because tuning into your body's natural circadian rhythm will help you balance out your insulin levels.

2. Avoid stimulants. Stimulants like caffeine and nicotine can take up to 8 hours to wear off completely. If you're one of those people who need a 3:00pm cup of coffee to help you get through the rest of the work day, consider having that cup of coffee at 1:00pm instead.

3. Don't take naps late in the day. Taking naps after 2:00 or 3:00 PM can make it harder to fall asleep when bedtime rolls around. If you need a nap, try to take it as early as possible. Try a 10 minute savasana (the corpse pose you do at the end of most yoga classes) instead.

4. Your bedroom is for sleeping — keep it that way. Having gadgets like your cell phone or a TV in your bedroom can be detrimental to your sleep. Keeping distractions like these completely out of the bedroom is a great way to ensure you fall asleep shortly after your head hits the pillow.

5. If you can't fall asleep, don't lie awake in bed. You likely will start getting anxious and worried when you can't fall asleep quickly. Your bed should be a relaxing place, so take your worries into another room and engage in a relaxing activity. Journal or make a to do list for tomorrow. Once your worries are on paper, you can rest easy. Once you start feeling sleepy, head back to bed.

BONUS TIP: Stay away from screens before bed. Find a bedtime routine that is relaxing and calming without the use of computers, phones or TV. Try a calming tea (chamomile or lemon balm), read a book, do some yoga poses, or wrap up household chores like dishes or laundry.

Bottomline:

Getting good quality sleep can help with hormone regulation, blood sugar, and weight loss. It's a basic need that must be met and also helps set you up for success with your new daily habits.

CHAPTER 9

Stress and Movement

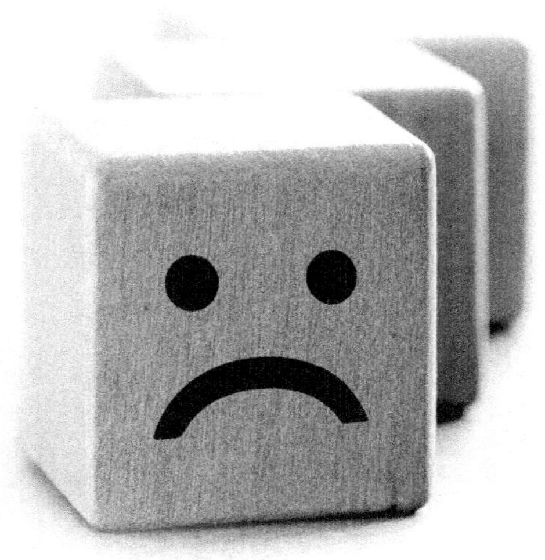

What is the secret MAJOR root cause of high blood sugar?

Answer: Stress

Let's take a serious moment to look at stress and how it impacts your body:

- Stress decreases your body's ability to produce stomach acid to breakdown and digest food.
- It can stop the "cleansing waves" in your gut that clean up after you eat, leaving unwanted bacteria there.
- It disrupts sleep and hormones and can cause you to feel tired during the day and "wired" at night. This is also why you see your blood sugar go up with stress.
- It weakens the immune system so it's less capable of fighting off invaders.

Stress not only impacts us physically, but also mentally and emotionally. When things in life start spiraling out of control, your body releases hormones to help you get through it. I'm sure you've heard of the body's "fight or flight" response. When faced with a "fight or flight" situation, your body releases cortisol and adrenaline into the bloodstream to amp you up in order to deal with whatever is happening to you. While all this is occurring, insulin levels decrease and your liver starts releasing sugar into the body. This is your reserve sugar when unexpected "dangerous" situations arise. As your cortisol and other hormone levels rise, insulin doesn't work as well, making your blood sugar go higher.

If you were truly running for your life, this would be a great response — but not when it occurs often or daily. If you operate in "flight or fight" mode for too long, year after year, it can fast forward your progression toward diabetes.

Oftentimes a go-to for managing stress is alcohol. A glass of wine or bottle of beer signifies calm, peace, and me-time for some. Alcohol as a symbol of "this is what I deserve for a crazy day", can quickly spiral out of control. Drinking alcohol regularly for stress management can do the following:

- Reduce sensitivity to insulin (resulting in high blood sugar)
- Decrease sleep quality
- Increase triglyceride level, which can increase risk of heart attack
- Heavy drinking can increase risk of pancreatitis, which can lead to diabetes
- Displacement and depletion of key nutrients that your body needs
- Possible interactions with other herbs, supplements, and medications, potentially causing low blood sugar reaction
- Damage to gut bacteria

Enjoying wine, beer, or spirits on occasion can be part of healthy living. Relying on alcohol for stress management can be very detrimental to health.

Real Life Stress

You met my mom, Beth, earlier. Let's take a look at how stress impacted her progression toward diabetes and perhaps you can relate.

She was in her early sixties when life as she knew it was upended. She and her husband had to temporarily move from their retirement home in the desert back to the Midwest to care for ailing parents. She and her husband wanted to care for her father-in-law in his home for as long as they could to help him maintain his independence. Her mother-in-law had passed away and her father-in-law had Alzheimer's and could no longer live alone nor adequately care for himself.

During this time, my mom lost a lot of control over her life. She couldn't always eat the meals she wanted; she couldn't always get out and do the walking she wanted. Life was unpredictable and she felt like almost everything was out of her control. She was not in her own space and her routine was very different and stressful. They spent the next few years caring for her ailing father-in-law in his home. She missed her retirement life and her own home. She was thankful to be there with and for her husband in caring for her father-in-law, but caring for a loved one in this capacity was not something she was prepared for. Her stress level was running at max for an extended period of time. This was when she was diagnosed with prediabetes.

Everyone has to deal with stress from time to time. It's an unavoidable part of life. Some people don't deal with it very well. Many people enter their senior years expecting to retire and relax when life suddenly throws them a curveball and their plans are upended. When the body undergoes stress for extended periods, many of the body's systems become worn down and fatigued. Think about a wild animal being hunted. When that animal senses danger, "fight or flight" hormones kick in and the animal is in pure survival mode.

Human beings are not meant to function in "fight or flight" mode every day. Particularly at mealtime, we need to be able to rest and digest. Can you imagine trying to feed this hunted animal while it's running for its life? Can you imagine the fatigue this animal would feel if it was never able to feel safe and secure? Its lifespan would likely be limited. Stress needs to be taken seriously.

Stress can account for some extreme spikes in blood sugar. I've observed many of my client's continuous glucose monitoring graphs and seen spikes of 50+ mg/dl – all related to stress. Whether it's due to news, phone calls with family members, or just an isolated stressful life event, no one is immune to the impact of stress. The way stress is dealt with, however, is within our control.

I had a client who exercised 3 days per week, was a vegetarian and ate high quality food. She had a stressful event one evening and her blood sugar spiked from 94mg/dl to 154mg/dl. She did not have diabetes, only prediabetes, and still her blood sugar spiked over 50 points from a stressful event!

What is one of the most underutilized tools we have to deal with stress?

I bet you thought I was going to say exercise! While exercise is important and we will definitely talk about it, we first need to address the way we breathe.

There are a lot of different ways to breathe. When we're stressed, we tend to breathe very shallow from our chest rather than taking deep belly breaths. Since breathing is something we can control and do anytime, anywhere, it is a useful tool for managing stress. When you're under stress, there are times during the day when you may feel run down and low on energy, and other times when you feel revved up. Here are some different breathing techniques to help you in either situation.

The stimulating breath:

This one is great for increasing energy and alertness, especially during that 3pm slump. Try it when you wake up in the morning, when you get that coffee or sugar craving in the afternoon or before a workout. It also benefits those with depression or anxiety.

Here is how you do it:

- Find a comfortable seated position. Connect the tip of your thumb to the tip of your index finger and hold your other fingers straight. Let the back of your hands rest on your knees or lap.
- Breathe in and out only through your nose (this one is called Bhastrika, also known as Bellows breath). This breath actually comes from the chest and the belly expanding. It's beneficial to add your arms into this practice as well.
- As you inhale through your nose, reach your arms to the sky with open palms. Notice your belly expanding or pushing out. As you exhale through your nose, pull your arms down and make a fist. Notice your belly pulling in. Inhale with the same force that you exhale. Each breath is quick.
- This isn't the quietest breathing you will ever do, but it's very effective at reenergizing and waking you up. You don't even have to do the arm movement in order for it

to be effective. Try a round for 10 breaths to start, then take a break for 30 seconds.

- Next try 20 breaths with another 30 second break. Finally try 30 breaths followed by several rounds of a slower breath to cool down.

You can experience more practice and guidance on this type of breathing by joining an online or in-person yoga class. Avoid this type of breathing if you ate within the last couple hours, are pregnant, have uncontrolled high blood pressure or suffer from seizures.

The 4-7-8 breathing exercise:

This breathing pattern was developed by Dr. Andrew Weil. Use this form of breath anytime you need to feel more calm and relaxed. It's especially effective if you do this daily, aiming for 4 breath cycles. It's a nice technique if you find yourself in the kitchen with food cravings.

- Start with the tip of your tongue placed on the roof of your mouth, behind your front teeth.
- Exhale completely with an open mouth and pursed lips.
- Close your mouth and inhale through your nose as you count in your head to "4", as your belly pushes out.
- Hold your breath in for a count of "7."
- Open mouth/pursed lips, tip of tongue on roof of mouth,

exhale all your air out for a count of "8," as the belly pulls in. You'll make a "whoosh" sound. Do a few rounds of this.

Alternate nostril breathing (Nadi Shodhana):

This is good for reducing anxiety and relaxation. It can even benefit your heart and improve respiratory function. If you have never done this before, I recommend you watch a video first, take a yoga class, or have someone read this to you as you try it.

- Sit upright. Take your right hand "peace" fingers (index and middle finger), and place them together between your eyebrows.
- Exhale all of your air, then close off your right nostril with your thumb.
- Inhale through your left nostril, then close off the left nostril with your ring finger.
- Open the right nostril and exhale through your right nostril. Then inhale through the (same) right nostril.
- Close the right nostril with your thumb and exhale through the left nostril.

That is one round or breath cycle. Always finish with an exhale on the left side. Try doing it for one minute and eventually work your way up to 5 minutes or more.

It's best to do this when you have an empty stomach. This is a nice way to calm your body before a meal to help with relaxation and digestion.

Many studies show that yoga can help lower stress and decrease your levels of the stress hormone cortisol. Fasting and post-meal blood sugar can be reduced when these or other similar types of breathing exercises are performed regularly.

Movement

I just know that this is what you've been waiting for and I'm not going to hold back. I'm giving this to you straight — moving is <u>not</u> negotiable.

A minimum of 150 minutes each week is recommended for people with diabetes. 300 minutes a week is recommended if you've lost a significant amount of weight and want to keep it off. But wait — don't slam the book shut just yet. I promise moving can be fun and that you will get to a point where it is the highlight of your day. You don't have to start with 150 minutes a week; you can gradually work your way up.

Can you start with 11 minutes a day? A recent study in ***British Journal of Sports Medicine*** showed us we need at least 11 minutes of daily exercise to live longer and counteract our typical 8 to 11 hours of sitting each day.

Simple ways to get started:

- Take a brisk walk. Bike ride for 11 minutes.
- Choose 6–10 different exercise moves and do each for 1–2 minutes (high knee march, jumping jacks, squats, jog in place, burpees, stair climb, ice skate, fast feet)
- Stop at a school track or trail on the way home from work and walk for 11 minutes. You just need good shoes and don't even have to change clothes.
- Take family members to the park and play tag, basketball, frisbee or walk around while they play.

Get creative, try anything that will get you moving and your heart pumping. If you are not familiar with some of the moves listed above, do a little research on the internet or make up your own.

Remember Norm? He didn't do any exercise for at least 6 weeks when we started working together. He then started with 5–15 minutes per session but was not consistent at first. Then he progressed to 15 minutes every day, and continued to bump it up by 5 minutes every week or so. He is now at 35+ minutes every single day. Do the math: that's 245 minutes a week! He also has an average blood sugar in the 120s now when it used to average around 220mg/dl. His A1c is now at 6%.

Let's take a look at the top 7 biggest misconceptions people have when it comes to exercise:

1. "I'm busy so that means I'm active." Be real with yourself. When you get to the end of your day, how many steps did you really take? I'm sure you were busy, but most of us don't get as much exercise as we need from daily activities alone. Any and all movement is great, but ask yourself how you can increase your daily movement from what you are already doing. The results you are getting with your current "dose" of exercising may not be cutting it.

2. Thinking it's "all or nothing". Some people think they have to spend 45-60 minutes for it to count as exercise. Well that's just not the case. Five minutes counts ... just do something, anything. You don't even need to put on special clothes. Just moving is enough to impact your blood sugar.

3. Treating exercise like it's something other people do. It's not. It's something YOU can do! It's non-negotiable because it is one of the most powerful prescriptions for diabetes. Create that vision of the "future you" and include a fun daily activity that requires movement.

4. Same thing, different day. Change it up! Sure you can take your daily walk but take a different route, stop avoiding that hill, pick up your pace...keep your body guessing.

5. Thinking that there is a BEST time to exercise. The BEST time is when you'll do it. Some people need to pop right out of bed and get to it; others prefer a midday workout. Think about when you have the most energy, when you can make the time, and when the least distractions and barriers will pop up.

6. Expecting it to be miserable. Exercise should be fun and enjoyable and, if it's not, you're doing it wrong! Pick 3 things that sound fun to do for movement or you might be interested in trying and write them down. Here are some ideas: martial arts/boxing, swimming, dancing, walking, biking, yoga/pilates, weights, group fitness classes, apps with workout classes, high intensity interval training, chair exercises, pickleball, volleyball, basketball, hockey. There are so many options. You can also pair something you really enjoy (such as music, movies, or audio books) with something you don't mind doing – like walking.

7. Being scared of what will happen if you start. Many people are afraid of low blood sugars, soreness, getting injured, or not doing it right/being embarrassed. Reach out to your healthcare team, share your concerns and come up with a safe plan for exercise.

Remember the acronym **FITT**. There are things you can alter to continue seeing results. For example, you might increase how hard you work while exercising, but decrease the time. You might keep your walks to 30 minutes, but add an extra day. Keep it interesting, mix it up. Don't let your body get too efficient and don't let your brain get bored!

F - Frequency. How often are you exercising? Can you increase from 3 days a week to 4 days?

I - Intensity. Can you make your heart beat faster on some days, slower on others? Changing your intensity can help you increase endurance.

T - Time. Maybe you start with 10 minutes. Over time, can you increase to 15 or 20+ minutes?

T - Type. It's great to find something you love, but can you change it up a little? Maybe you love walking, but could you try biking or dancing, or adding in some weights?

CHAPTER 10

What Technology Tools Will Help Me Monitor the Reversal of Diabetes?

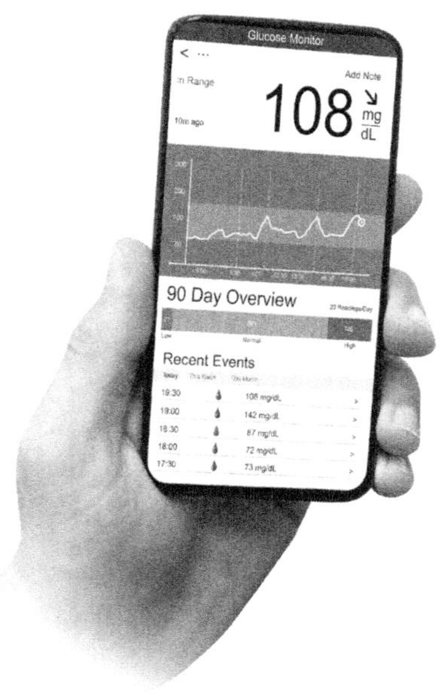

Look, I know sticking needles into your body is less than desirable. I'll lay that out there straight away. But here's the deal - the joy and satisfaction you feel when you see that number change based on your own actions is one of the best feelings because now you are in control. Day after day, clients will report what makes their blood sugar drop quickly or what makes it rise, yet they never would have been able to determine that without the ability to check blood sugar.

Yes, I explain to them that exercise can lower blood sugar and that certain foods will raise blood sugar more quickly than others — but seeing is believing. Feedback is an absolutely necessary motivating factor in reversing diabetes. Don't think for a second that you're checking your blood sugar for your doctor or for your diabetes educator. No. Absolutely not. Those numbers are for you.

You might be wondering — ***how often do I need to check my blood sugar?*** The answer is — ***that it is completely up to you***. You should check your blood sugar as often as you need to have that information, so get curious. You also may be wondering — if I have prediabetes, do I need to check? That answer is a little trickier but, in short, yes. Health insurance is not going to pay for a blood sugar meter for you if you have prediabetes. It will be an out-of-pocket expense, but you can find some reasonably-priced meters to purchase. Don't invest a lot in a blood sugar meter if you don't have diabetes. It's just a temporary tool to give you some feedback and once you get the information you need and you've successfully reversed your prediabetes, you will no longer need the meter on a daily basis.

Here are some reasons people check their blood sugar and when:

REASON TO CHECK	WHEN TO CHECK	WHY?
Exercise	Consider checking before you start and when you're done.	Most moderate cardio will help to lower blood sugar, but if you are racing, doing something more intense, or weight-lifting, you may see a temporary rise in blood sugar. This is OK. Exercise overall has a very powerful effect on the body, so don't panic if it goes up or down. Just gather information so you understand.
Vitamins/ Supplements/ Medication	Consider checking first thing in the morning before you eat or drink anything (water is OK). Check 2 hours after a meal.	If you start taking a pill to help lower blood sugar, it's important to make sure that pill is working, regardless of whether it's a medication or a supplement. You need to know what works well and what doesn't work.
Insulin	If you are taking a long-acting insulin, the best time to check is after a long period of fasting, and that is usually when you wake up.	You are checking to make sure the dose is right. If you get low blood glucose overnight, then your dose is likely too high.

REASON TO CHECK	WHEN TO CHECK	WHY?
Stress	Check randomly throughout the day when you are feeling stressed	This will let you see how high your blood sugar is going and give you the opportunity to take immediate action, such as deep breathing or taking a leisurely walk to calm down.
Sick/Illness	Check randomly throughout the day	When you are sick, your blood sugar can go high and, if it goes high and stays high, you will want to check in with your healthcare provider. On the flip side, if you are sick and are taking medications but can't eat, you may see it drop low. Note that if you are prescribed steroids for an illness, it can cause your blood sugar to go high.

TIME OF DAY	BLOOD SUGAR TARGET GOALS TO REVERSE DIABETES	BLOOD SUGAR TARGET GOALS TO CONTROLDIABETES
Wake up (fasting)	70-110 mg/dl	80-130 mg/dl
2 hours after eating	<140 mg/dl	<160-180 mg/dl
Bedtime	<120 mg/dl	<140 mg/dl

Note: Make sure you communicate with your team to let them know your goals so they can help you come up with a safe plan to get there. Blood sugar and A1c goals are individualized, just like your eating style.

OK, so we've talked about the importance of knowing what your blood sugar is day to day; we've talked about when to check and also reviewed what your target goals are. Now we need to talk about how to get this information. There are several options when it comes to monitoring your blood sugar. My favorite option for everyone is a continuous glucose monitor (CGM).

At the time of publication of this book, the cheapest and most accessible CGM is the Freestyle Libre brand by Abbott. There are already various versions of this CGM but, even if your insurance doesn't cover it, your healthcare provider could write you a prescription for it. Paying for one out of pocket could be perfectly feasible. I have no connection with Abbott, the company that makes the Libre – I just happen to like it a lot, particularly for people with type 2 diabetes. It currently doesn't have alerts and alarms but that is in progress. There are many very good CGMs on the market.

The reason CGM is superior to single finger sticks is that you are able to see a moving picture of everything that happened during your day. It's kind of like watching a video of an event versus just seeing a few pictures someone took of the event.

Finger sticks are the snapshots and CGM is the video. With that said, if for some reason you cannot get access to a CGM, finger sticks will still give you some great data, so don't despair.

There are also apps available for people with diabetes who are looking to house all of their diabetes information in one place. They are constantly changing, but here are some long-standing apps:

NAME OF THE APP	WHAT IT DOES
My Sugr (iOS and Android) free version.	Personalized logging, overview progress report, estimated HbA1c, insulin calculator in pro version, and pings you reminders if you choose. Works best with Accu check blood sugar meters.
Glooko	Connects you with your provider so you have better communication about your diabetes
Diabetes: M	Fingerstick reminders, food logging, integrates with fitness apps, blood sugar trend mapping, insulin bolus calculator based on the nutritional information you add.
Tidepool	A great way to upload your device and connect with your healthcare provider.
Glucose Companion	Track all your metrics including blood sugar and weight. If you don't have a CGM, this is helpful as it will report weekly graphs with averages.

NAME OF THE APP	WHAT IT DOES
Glucose Buddy	Tracks blood glucose, medication, meals, and track trends, has a food database (can scan barcodes), syncs to the Dexcom CGM and Apple Health app to track your steps and other physical activity. Can export data to printable reports. It also includes a 12-week diabetes education that features five-minute lessons.

Bottomline:

You have heard a few stories in the previous chapters of people who have used a continuous glucose monitor. The data they received was invaluable and life-changing. The apps are a nice way to keep your diabetes team connected and save you time and trouble when it comes to getting your data to your team. Find something that works for you and allows you to track and record key factors such as food, medications, supplements, exercise, life events/stress and - of course - your blood sugar.

CHAPTER 11

Putting It All Together

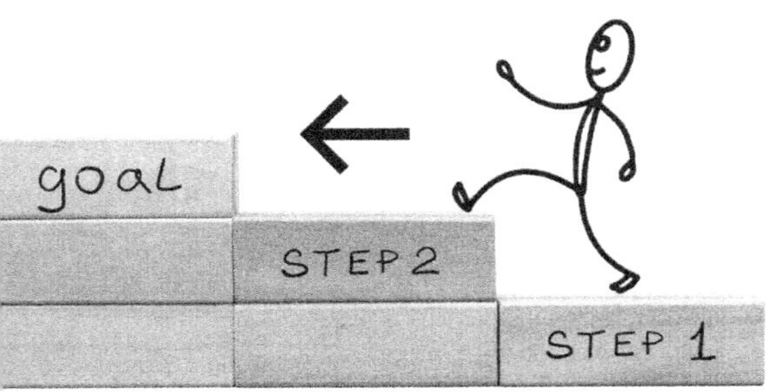

DIABETES →

Allow me to introduce you to Susan. She has had type 2 diabetes for the last 15 years. Her mom also had diabetes and took insulin for many years. Susan remembers always wanting her mom to eat healthier. It pained her to see her mom buying danishes and donuts, but her mom never listened when she tried to convince her to make healthier choices. They were very close; they did everything together. Much of what they did revolved around food. They loved to run errands and eat out. Eventually, Susan's mom passed away and the loss was devastating.

As time went on, Susan would phase in and out between checking her blood sugar and trying to make healthy changes. However, she just couldn't seem to be consistent. The commitment wasn't there. Deep down, she feared losing her favorite foods, her pastime of eating out, and her love of cooking and baking. Eventually, she met with a diabetes educator and began making some changes. With a few small changes such as walking, not drinking soda and snacking less, she noticed immediate results. At each doctor visit she would see a little improvement in her lab tests. Her doctor wanted to add medication but she would negotiate and say "just give me three more months." During that three months, something would always come up to throw her off track, like a trip or family event.

Eventually she was on insulin, metformin, jardiance, and Victoza, and her lifestyle changes regressed. Susan stopped exercising, her blood sugar went higher, and she started to notice her weight increasing. She was beginning to follow in her mother's footsteps. Although Susan could clearly see the problem with her mom's behavior and the cause of her high blood sugar, denial prevented Susan from taking action to reverse her own diabetes. Not only is diabetes genetic but its inherent emotional trauma is passed down as history repeats itself.

When someone is in denial, there is little you can do to change them. All you can do is be there and support them. Telling your loved ones what they should or shouldn't be doing typically doesn't create that "aha" moment of truth and it can sometimes cause more spite. For some, it's a wake-up call when they hear it from a healthcare provider they respect. Or it's using some sort of technology like a continuous glucose monitor or a simple blood sugar meter to see the cause and effect related to their blood sugar. And unfortunately for others, it's a catastrophic health event that brings on urgency to make changes. Taking charge of one's health is a personal decision that comes from an "aha" moment which leads to a strong "why."

Unfortunately, not everyone has that "aha" moment, but it's definitely not too late for you. The underlying factor here is usually emotions, whether it's sadness, anger, frustration, or fear – not necessarily fear of complications but fear that their "joy" in life is getting taken away. I'll often hear people say, "if it tastes good, it must be bad for you." So now eating healthful, high-quality food is looked upon as a punishment and many people are fearful that their joy of food will be removed and they will have nothing.

Even if you aren't fully convinced that making these changes are right for you, you can still choose some small steps to get you moving in the right direction. Even if you don't do an overhaul of your diet, you can still make some other changes that won't upend your life. Instead of focusing on taking things away, perhaps pick some foods you read about that could be of benefit and start incorporating them into meals.

Remember this: diabetes is living within you and <u>you</u> call the shots on how to deal with it. Will you choose to ignore and deny or will you acknowledge and find harmony with diabetes?

If you are supporting a loved one, the best way to help is to lead by example. Make or order healthful food when you are together, invite them to do something active with you, and be there to listen rather than constantly giving advice. It's hard, particularly when that person is near and dear to you – but each of us is responsible for our own health and decisions in life.

If you are the one living with diabetes and you constantly have loved ones telling you what to do, think about it from their perspective. Truly, they are not trying to hurt or torture you. They likely care deeply for you and are trying to help. Have a straightforward conversation with them on how they can best support you and let them know what "help" you prefer that they may not be providing.

We can choose to face diabetes head on and use the tools we have in our toolbox to start a journey, whereby living in harmony with diabetes is the destination. Or we can pretend it's not there and ignore it completely until it wreaks havoc and prevents us from living life the way we intended.

Surround yourself with people who care about you and can support you. Touch base with a counselor to talk about some of your concerns. Find a diabetes educator for support, regardless of where you are in your process of taking steps to prevent or reverse diabetes. If you've accepted that diabetes is within you, then surround yourself with a team that can help you take charge and live in harmony with it.

Step 1: Acknowledge diabetes

Acknowledge that diabetes is part of your life and that you can live in harmony with it. Diabetes does not have to take away everything and everyone that you love.

Step 2: Believe in yourself

Know that what you do matters. This is not a hopeless situation; small changes can have monumental results.

Step 3: Trust the process

Trust that your "aha" moment will come and, when it does, there is no turning back!

Earlier, I spoke of Benjamin Hardy, PhD, the organizational psychologist who helps people reset their thinking to accomplish big goals. I find him fascinating and motivating. He talks a lot about envisioning your future self. We are constantly evolving — sometimes achieving important growth and sometimes regressing. Once you're able to start wrapping your mind around what you want, you can then start reverse-engineering what it takes to get there. Picture yourself doing things that bring you the health status and joy that you want to experience in life.

You manage what you measure. Each week, hold yourself accountable by listing your goals and then rating yourself at the end of the week on how you did. Reflect on why things went well (or didn't). Creating and reviewing a list of goals that align with your priorities will help you achieve your goals, and ensure that they remain in the forefront.

We touched on mindfulness early in the book but focused mainly on being mindful while eating. Imagine if mindfulness was integrated into all parts of your life. Mindfulness is being present in the moment. When you're out for a walk or hike, try enjoying your surroundings rather than thinking about just getting it over with so you can move on with the next thing. Take time to make eye contact with a friend or family member as you spend time together. Recognize how your body feels when your blood sugar is 250mg/dl 100mg/dl. The more mindfulness is present in our lives, the easier it is to become the person we want to be and attain the optimal health that we long for.

The key here is focusing on one small step at a time and taking it all in. Don't rush it. I know high blood sugar can feel like an emergency and you want to overhaul every aspect of your life to get rid of it (or completely ignore it and pretend it's not happening), but take time to savor the lessons learned in each step. Be mindful and observant with each step you take toward your future self. Savor each new attempt on this journey to change. See how far you can take it and how far you have come. With every small step, you are getting closer to your future self while distancing yourself from the effects of diabetes. Just keep going.

The steps to putting it all together

Here is a recap of what we know can help to reverse the path to diabetes. I'm not promising diabetes will disappear, but you can take steps in the opposite direction and here is how:

5 Rs	CONSIDERATIONS TO OUTSMART YOUR DIABETES
REMOVE	Food, stress, infections, toxins (chemicals, metals, thoughts, behaviors), sedentary lifestyle. Some antimicrobials may be needed here to get rid of any underlying "good bacteria killers" living in the gut. In this phase we are "weeding out" the garden, so the good stuff has room to grow.
REPLACE	Add high quality food, digestive help (chewing more, bitters, assess need for Betaine HCL), sleep, activity, assess need for CoQ10 (especially if on statin) and other nutrient deficiencies. Food sources of CoQ10: Organ meats, pork, beef, chicken, fatty fish, spinach, cauliflower, broccoli, oranges, strawberries, soybeans, lentils, peanuts, sesame seeds and pistachios.
REINOCULATE	High fiber food and resistant starch, targeted probiotics/prebiotics, fermented foods (for some)
REPAIR	Bone broth, L-glutamine, Vitamins A, C, & D with K2-MK7, Zinc, Magnesium, Arginine, Alpha Lipoic Acid, EPA/DHA, Quercetin, Choline, and other powerful antioxidants. Further gut repair: Slippery Elm, DGL, Marshmallow, Colostrum, Curcumin Acupuncture or other modalities such as massage to improve circulation and manage stress. Note: all of these are not necessary, it should be individualized
REBALANCE	Making choices in line with your priorities and future self, having time for rest and fun. Incorporate breathing, meditation, or any mindful movement. Increasing daily movement and getting at least 20 minutes daily of moderate/vigorous activity. Continue to monitor blood sugar as a way to feel confident that your plan is working. Find a team of support people to help you stay on track (friend, family, healthcare provider/Certified Diabetes Care and Education Specialist).

Tips for everything you learned:

- **Fasting:** 12–16 hours of fasting to let your body reset and repair. This can also be beneficial for improving insulin resistance and heart health. This is easily done after dinner and while you sleep. Decide if it's a tool that will work for you.
- **Food as medicine prescription:** 2–3 cups of leafy greens (spinach, kale, arugula, chard, etc), 2–3 cups of colorful fruits and vegetables, 2–3 cups of cruciferous, sulfur-rich vegetables (broccoli, cabbage, cauliflower, Brussels sprouts, bok choy etc). These vegetables can be more powerful than medication when it comes to reversing inflammation. Start with one cup from each group and work your way up.
- **Fiber.** Focusing on fruits and vegetables should help get you to your target goal of 30+ grams of dietary fiber per day to help with reversing diabetes. Fiber helps you feel full. It also helps clean up and clear out what doesn't need to be in the body. Resistant starch feeds friendly bacteria.
- **Protein.** Know where your protein came from and what it ate (grass-fed, organic, wild caught). You deserve the best. Put high-quality food in your body.
- **Try new things.** Don't eat the exact same food over and over. My best tip here is to be adventurous. If you go out to a nice restaurant, be willing to try a new food,

particularly a vegetable dish or salad that you wouldn't normally get. Chefs are amazing, so give them a chance to show you how good, quality food can really taste when prepared properly. You might even consider taking a cooking class. Eat food that is in season.

- **Eat just enough.** Let your body guide you. Be present at mealtimes, eat in a designated place, take a deep breath, chew slowly, and enjoy. No more measuring out restricting portions of food and counting calories. Put a little on your plate to start. You can always have seconds if you are still hungry. Just prioritize which food will nourish both your body and mind and eat when you have the physical feeling to do so.
- **Weekly meal planning and prep.** Wouldn't it be amazing if food just appeared on the table when you're hungry? I dream about this every day! It turns out that the only way meals appear is if I plan, prep, and serve it. What day of the week will you do your meal prep and planning?
- **Keep a daily journal.** Begin each day by writing your intentions for that day, what you will focus on and accomplish, and how you will make sure it happens. At the end of the day, what kind of results did you get?
- **Sleep.** Rest and repair of the body is important. How can you set up a routine to make sure you are getting 7-9 hours of sleep each night? Having a good go-to-bed plan and a solid wake-up plan can set you up for

success for the rest of the day. Four hours won't cut it if you are not sleeping well. A change in diet and a change in daily activities can help. Talk to your provider or educator. Sleeping pills are not the answer. See what you can change in your environment to improve your sleep.

- **Environment.** Is your environment set-up in a way so that the "easy" choice is the "healthy" choice? What is easily accessible to eat at home or work? Set-up "speed bumps" to throw you off the track of old habits. Move common snack foods to a new location to give you a pause. Eat your snacks off a plate at the table with no distractions and see if the food is still as desirable.
- **Stress.** What are you dealing with and how are you dealing with it? What strategy did you choose to help you manage your stress? A reminder that this is one of the biggest factors driving people toward diabetes. Really think about how you can incorporate breathing, meditation, and/or yoga into your daily life. Managing stress can put the brakes on diabetes.
- **Friends.** Your inner circle of people, the ones you spend the majority of your time with should have values similar to yours. If you find that your inner circle is not aligning with the values of your future self, make adjustments accordingly. Change is inevitable. It doesn't mean you can't be friends anymore but are your influencers the people you're closest to? Are they

helping you to live the life of your future self and reverse diabetes?

- **Joy vs Junk.** Cleaning up your environment helps relieve anxiety and can improve your health, both mentally and physically. Start one drawer or closet at a time. Get rid of things that don't serve you anymore, much like you are ridding your life of old behaviors that no longer serve you. Toss out the old to make space for what is most important.
- **Movement.** Be sure to take time weekly to include a variety of activities that serve you. Focus on improving strength, cardiovascular function, flexibility, and endurance. Vary your intensity. Continue to challenge yourself. For those of you who like number goals, aim for a minimum of 150 minutes per week as your base dose of exercise. You can always increase the dose to 200–300 minutes a week for further benefits.

In closing, I hope you have been enlightened and inspired by the information, thoughts and suggestions I've shared with you. You are an individual and your eating style should reflect that fact. I encourage you to continue making time for yourself each week — to check your goals, acknowledge your progress, and pinpoint what needs to change. This is an ongoing process and I hope you will never, never, never give up as you pursue better health. Expect to change and evolve as you move step-by-step toward your future self. May you achieve your every goal and always enjoy the journey!

Angela Manderfeld RD

APPENDIX

The resources below will help you work through the exercises in the book and create your individualized eating style. For free printable versions of the Carbohydrate Guide, Foods High in Dietary Fiber, 5 R Plan for Diabetes, Step-by-Step Eating Style Worksheet and GF Anti-Inflammatory Food List please visit www.outsmartyourdiabetes.com/oyd-extras.

Additional Resources:

Helpful shopping tips, meal prep and recipe ideas:
www.100daysofrealfood.com

Meal plans created by registered dietitians
https://outsmartyourdiabetes.com/products/

Help with creating your "future self"

https://benjaminhardy.com/

Breathing Techniques

https://www.drweil.com/videos-features/videos/breathing-exercises-4-7-8-breath/

Carbohydrate Guide

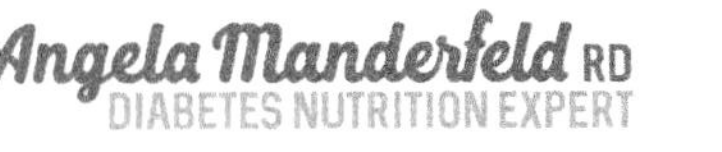

OUTSMART YOUR DIABETES

Carbohydrate Guide

The goal of this guide is to raise awareness about quality and quantity of carbohydrates. They are a very important part of our diet and should not be excluded.

Food Category	Each serving to the left contains....	Helpful Hints:
NON- STARCHY VEGETABLES		
Artichoke, asparagus, boy chow, green beans, broccoli, cabbage, carrots, cauliflower, celery, cucumber, greens, mushroom, okra, onions, pea pods, peppers, salad greens, spinach, summer squash, tomato, zucchini	1c raw or 1/2 cup cooked is **~5 grams of carbs per serving**	Try to fill half of you plate with these! Only 5 grams of carbohydrate per serving. This group contains a LOT of FIBER. Vegetables will help you feel full after a meal. Cover half of your plate with them! Aim for 2 servings at each meal. These also make great snacks if you need one.
STARCHY VEGETABLES & BEANS		
Beans, corn, lentils, peas, potato, yam, sweet potato **1/2 c** Lima beans **2/3 c** Winter Squash, mixed veg **1c**	**~15g carbs per serving**	Beans typically have about 4-7 g fiber per 1/2 cup! These vegetables also have good fiber content. Aim for 25-40g of dietary fiber each day! The more fiber you eat, the easier it is to stabilize blood sugar and lose weight.
GRAINS		
1 oz slice bread/bagel, **1/2** bun Rice, Pasta **1/3 c cooked** Oats, Grits **1/2c cooked** Tortilla, pita **6 in** Waffle, pancake **4 in**	**~15g carbs per serving**	Choose high quality cereals, breads, etc. Read the ingredients, look for whole grains and lots of fiber. Oatmeal is my favorite cereal choice. Avoid granola unless you very carefully read the label, look for no added sugar, and use granola as a topper/side, rather than your entire meal.

Download free printable version at www.outsmartyourdiabetes.com/oyd-extras

Carbohydrate Guide - CONTINUED

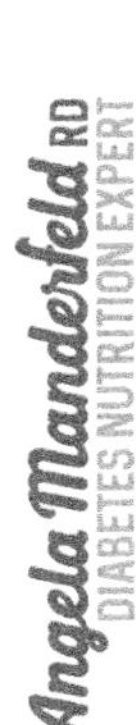

OUTSMART YOUR DIABETES

MILK, YOGURT		
Cow's Milk, Soy milk, Buttermilk, Goat's milk **1 cup** Plain Almond milk **1 cup** Plain Yogurt **6 oz.**	**~11-15g carbs per serving**	Yogurt has probiotics, so if you are lactose intolerant, you may tolerate yogurt in small amounts. The live, active cultures are good for your gut health. You can also find a variety of non-dairy alternatives if needed.
FRUIT		
Apple, banana, peach, orange - **1 small** Honeydew or cantaloupe cubes, raspberries, strawberries, watermelon **~1cup to 1 1/4 cup** Pineapple, blackberries, blueberries - **3/4 cup**	**~15 grams carbs**	Avoid juices as they do not have any fiber and they cause a quick rise in blood sugar which can zap energy. Exceptions here are if you are an athlete and are needing to increase your carbohydrate intake. Otherwise, juice should be avoided or limited; choose the whole fruit instead. A "small" fruit is about 4-6 oz. or the size of a tennis ball. Berries are high in fiber and antioxidants Aim for at least 2 fruit servings a day.
SWEETS		
Honey, Jam/Jelly, Sugar 1 Tbsp Brownie/unfrosted cake square 2 in 2 small cookies	**15 grams carbs**	These should be limited. Ideally no more than 6 tsps (24grams) of added sugar per day from women/kids, and no more than 9 tsps (36 grams) of added sugar per day for men. Too much can be an energy zapper....
ARTIFICIAL SWEETENERS		
Sucralose (splenda), Saccharin (Sweet n Low or Sugar Twin), Acesulfame Potassium (Ace-K, Sweet one, Swiss Sweet, Sunett), Advantame, Neotame. "Sugar Free" foods typically have sugar alcohols and sugar alcohols are not artificial, but partially resistant to digestion.	**use sparingly, if at all**	Stevia leaf extract or monk fruit are natural sweeteners, not artificial, these may be less risky options. Researchers have found that artificial sweeteners alter gut bacteria and make rodents more susceptible to glucose intolerance. The study subjects were not humans, but it's still worth paying attention to. My best advice is keep it as real as you can when it comes to nourishing your body. Less is definitely more when it comes to artificial sweeteners.

When reading a food label, first look at **Serving Size**, then **Total Carbohydrates** (for that serving), then fiber. Sugars are included in the total carbohydrates so don't add them up separately. Also, take a look at the ingredients and remember, less is more.

OutSmartYourDiabetes.com 2

Download free printable version at www.outsmartyourdiabetes.com/oyd-extras

5 R plan for diabetes

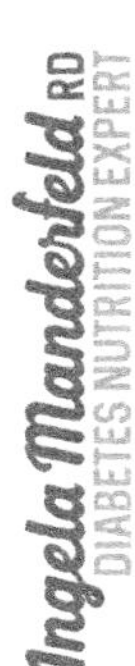

OUTSMART YOUR DIABETES

Outline for Reversing Diabetes

5 R's	Considerations
REMOVE	Food, stress, infections, toxins (chemicals, metals, thoughts, behaviors), sedentary lifestyle
REPLACE	High quality food, digestive help (chewing more, bitters, assess need for Betaine HCL), sleep, activity, assess need for CoQ10 (especially if on statin) and other nutrient deficiencies
REINOCULATE	High fiber food and resistant starch, targeted probiotics/prebiotics, fermented foods (for some)
REPAIR	Bone broth, L-glutamine, Vitamins A, C, & D, Zinc, Magnesium, Arginine, EPA/DHA, Quercetin, Choline, and other powerful antioxidants. Further gut repair: slippery elm, DGL, marshmallow, colostrum, curcumin Alpha lipoid acid for peripheral neuropathy Acupuncture or other modalities such as massage to improve circulation and manage stress. Note: not necessarily ALL of these are necessary, it should be individualized
REBALANCE	Making choices in line with your priorities and future self, having time for rest and fun. Incorporate breathing, meditation, or any mindful movement. Increasing daily movement and getting at least 20 minutes daily of moderate/vigorous activity. Continue to monitor blood sugar as a way to feel confident that your plan is working. Find a team of support people to help you stay on track (friend, family, healthcare provider/Certified Diabetes Care and Education Specialist).

Download free printable version at www.outsmartyourdiabetes.com/oyd-extras

5 R plan for diabetes - CONTINUED

Angela Manderfeld RD
DIABETES NUTRITION EXPERT

Outsmart your Diabetes

My 5-R Plan for Reversing Diabetes - Be specific.

5 R's	Details of my plan:
REMOVE	
REPLACE	
REINOCULATE	
REPAIR	
REBALANCE	

Download free printable version at www.outsmartyourdiabetes.com/oyd-extras

Foods High in Dietary Fiber

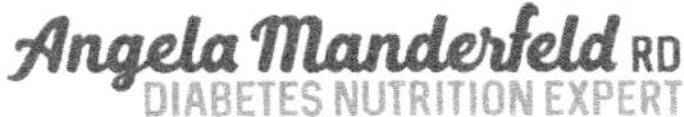

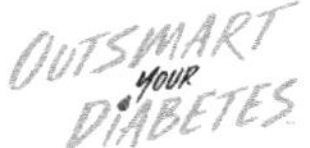

Foods High in Dietary Fiber

FOOD	SERVING SIZE	TOTAL FIBER
FRUITS		
Apple with skin	1 med apple	4.4
Banana	1 med banana	3.1
Oranges	1 med orange	3.1
Prunes	1 cup pitted	12.4
Raspberries	1 cup	8.0
Pear with skin	1 med pear	5.5
Strawberries, halves	1 cup	3.0
GRAINS, CEREALS, PASTA		
Spaghetti, whole wheat, cooked	1 cup	6.3
Barley, pearled, cooked	1 cup	6.0
Bran Flakes	3/4 cup	5.3
Oat bran muffin	1 medium	5.2
Oatmeal, instant, cooked	1 cup	4.0
Popcorn, air popped	3 cups	3.5
Brown Rice, cooked	1 cup	3.5
Whole wheat, multigrain, rye bread	1 slice	1.9

Source: USDA National Nutrient Database for Standard Reference, 2012

OutSmartYourDiabetes.com 1

Download free printable version at www.outsmartyourdiabetes.com/oyd-extras

Foods High in Dietary Fiber - CONTINUED

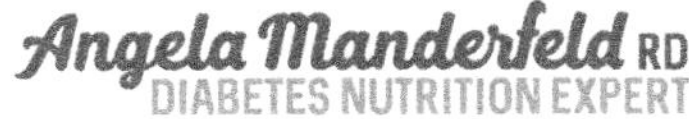

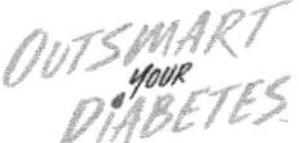

LEGUMES, NUTS, SEEDS		
Split peas, cooked	1 cup	16.3
Lentils, cooked	1 cup	15.6
Black beans, cooked	1 cup	15.0
Lima beans, cooked	1 cup	13.2
Baked beans, vegetarian, canned, cooked	1 cup	10.4
Sunflower seed kernels	1/4 cup	3.9
Almonds	1 oz (~23 nuts)	3.5
Pistachios	1 oz (~49 nuts)	2.9
Pecans	1 oz (19 halves)	2.7
VEGETABLES		
Artichoke, cooked	1 medium	10.3
Green peas, cooked	1 cup	8.8
Broccoli, steamed	1 cup	5.1
Turnip Greens, steamed	1 cup	5.0
Brussels Sprouts, cooked	1 cup	4.1
Sweet corn, cooked	1 cup	4.0
Potato with skin, baked	1 small	3.0
Carrot, raw	1 medium	1.7
Tomato	1 medium	1.5
Cucumber with peel	1 medium	1.5
Spinach	1 cup	0.7

Source: USDA National Nutrient Database for Standard Reference, 2012

OutSmartYourDiabetes.com 2

Download free printable version at www.outsmartyourdiabetes.com/oyd-extras

Step-by-Step Eating Style Worksheet

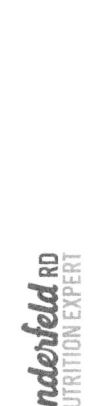

OUTSMART YOUR DIABETES

My Step by Step Individualized Plan Worksheet

FOOD CATEGORIES	My Individualized Eating Style - list the foods you like and are willing to try. These will be your core foods.(Refer to the book and other handouts if you are not sure what foods are included in each group)
Non Starchy Vegetables	
Starchy Vegetables, Grains, Beans	
Fruit	
Healthy Fats (nuts, seeds and oils)	
Protein	
Hydration/Drinks (ideally drinks with no calories, no artificial sweeteners)	
Foods I enjoy, not listed above. **(Make notes about if these foods are daily or weekly/monthly and if changing them to be higher quality would be beneficial)**	

The above food list can help you with grocery shopping and meal planning.

OutSmartYourDiabetes.com 1

Download free printable version at www.outsmartyourdiabetes.com/oyd-extras

Step-by-Step Eating Style Worksheet - CONTINUED

Angela Manderfeld RD
DIABETES NUTRITION EXPERT

OUTSMART YOUR DIABETES

TOOLS	List the approach or details you will take, with the tools listed in the left hand column.
Fasting: will I do this? If so, list fasting patterns that you will try. If no, leave blank.	
Meal planning help: Living Plate Meal Plans (see Angela's website), mealime (free app). Describe how you will plan your meals for the week. When will you do it and when will you shop? Who will do the meal prep/cooking?	
My Why? Take a moment to write down why these changes need to happen, refer to the book on how to drill this down. (see introduction in book for guidance)	
Daily Journal: What do you want to track? Examples: Goals for the day/week, blood sugar levels, blood pressure, what went well today, what did I learn today, how would I rate myself today/this week for staying on track with my goals, what got in my way, what makes my blood sugar go high, what doesn't?	

Step-by-Step Eating Style Worksheet - CONTINUED

Angela Manderfeld RD
DIABETES NUTRITION EXPERT

OUTSMART YOUR DIABETES

TOOLS	List the approach or details you will take, with the tools listed in the left hand column.
Technology: How will you track your blood sugar to see how your changes impact you? Get a blood sugar meter or continuous glucose monitor. You will need a prescription your provider for insurance to cover it. You will also need enough test strips while you are experimenting. I recommend asking for enough to do 4 fingersticks a day, to start. You can always back off later. What are your blood sugar goals (fasting/pre-meal, 2 hr after a meal, A1c goal)? (See introduction of book and Ch. 9)	
Sleep Routine: What do I need to do to improve my sleep habits? Stop screens an hour before bed, wind down with chamomile tea, read/meditate before bed, journal positives of the day/goals/ plan for tomorrow, cut off food a few hours before sleep, etc.	
Environment: Is there anything at home or at work that is setting me up for failure/sabotage. Focus on things you can control. Take actions to make the healthy choice the easy choice. (moving trigger foods to different location or out of the house, take candy jar off your desk, put meds in a place you will remember to take them, sit a glass on the counter to remind you to drink water, etc) Feel free to come up with your own.	

OutSmartYourDiabetes.com 3

Download free printable version at www.outsmartyourdiabetes.com/oyd-extras

Step-by-Step Eating Style Worksheet - CONTINUED

Angela Manderfeld RD
DIABETES NUTRITION EXPERT

OUTSMART YOUR DIABETES

Stress: How will you manage stress? Examples: exercise, breathing, meditation, hobby, support person, etc.	

TOOLS	List the approach or details you will take, with the tools listed in the left hand column.
What do I need more of (gives me energy), what do I need less of (drains me)? Think about people and possessions. Make sure you are allotting more time for the "energy" and less time for the "drains."	
Exercise as Medicine: Remember the FITT (frequency, intensity, time, type) rule. Daily movement is necessary, where in your day will you make time. Some days may be shorter sessions than others, but exercise is your medicine. What will you do? Plan your exercise for the week - day, time, what you will do, with who, and for how long. Schedule it.	When? What time? What will I do? How long? How will I hold myself accountable?
Medications/Supplements: Am I taking them as prescribed? If not, have I had a discussion with my provider about it. Is there a supplement or medication I think I need (have conversation with your provider)?	

Other Notes:

Download free printable version at www.outsmartyourdiabetes.com/oyd-extras

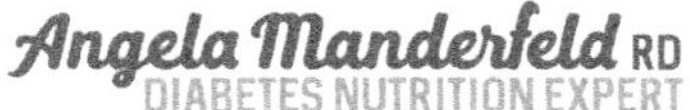

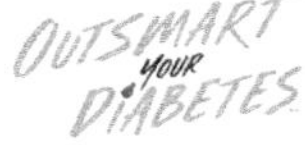

Anti-Inflammatory Eating Style

Gluten-Free

Before we can discuss what to eat, it's important to understand the following concepts.

QUALITY: You deserve the best. Don't compromise on your food, it's important to provide your body with the highest quality food. High quality food is your medicine. Low quality food causes inflammation

QUANTITY: Eat just enough. Optimal health is not about starving yourself, but it's about paying attention to cues to know when you are hungry or full. If you aren't getting these cues or you don't recognize them, eat half of what you normally would. You can always eat again later, but you need to cut back to realize how much you truly need. Avoid snacking until you start getting cues. Excess food causes inflammation.

DIVERSITY: It's easy to choose the same foods over and over. I'm not going to tell you to quit eating your favorite food, but see if you can add in some variety! By diversifying your food you're making sure you don't get too much of a good thing and you are also exposing your taste buds to different flavors and textures which can increase satisfaction. Also, when you are diverse within a meal and have a good balance of nutrients you may notice your energy improve and you feel satisfied for longer.

Circle or highlight the foods below that you enjoy eating or are willing to try.

GF Anti-Inflammatory Food List - CONTINUED

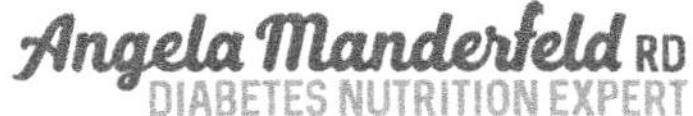

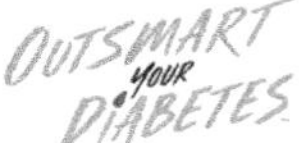

NON- STARCHY VEGETABLES	Artichokes, Asparagus, Bamboo shoots, Beans (green, wax, Italian) Bean sprouts, Beets, Brussels sprouts, Broccoli, Cabbage (green, bok choy, Chinese), Carrots Cauliflower, Celery, Cucumber, Eggplant Greens (collard, kale, mustard, turnip), Hearts of palm, Jicama, Kohlrabi, Leeks, Mushrooms, Okra, Onions, Pea Pods, Peppers, Radishes, Rutabaga, Salad Greens (endive, escarole, romaine, spinach, arugula, radicchio) Onions, Pea pods, Peppers, Radishes, Rutabaga, Sprouts, Squash (summer, spaghetti, zucchini) Sugar snap peas, Swiss chard, Tomato Turnips, Water chestnuts
GRAINS and STARCHY VEGETABLES	Amaranth, Buckwheat, Millet, Oats (certified), Rice, Quinoa, Sorghum, Teff Acorn squash, butternut squash, corn, green peas, parsnip, potatoes, pumpkin, sweet potatoes
BEANS, LENTILS, NUTS, SEEDS and PROTEIN	Black beans, chickpeas (garbanzo beans), soybeans, fava (broad) beans, kidney beans, lentils, lima beans, navy beans, pinto beans Almonds, brazil nuts, cashews, chestnut, hazelnut, peanuts, pecans, pine nut, pistacchio, macadamia, walnuts Chia, hemp, pumpkin, sesame, sunflower Chicken, eggs, fish, grass fed beef, pork, shellfish, wild game, dairy
FRUITS	Açaí, apple, apricot, avocado, banana, blackberry black currant, blueberry, cherry, coconut, cranberry, date Dragonfruit, elderberry, fig, grape, grapefruit, guava, jackfruit, kiwi, lemon, lime, lychee, mango, melon (cantaloupe, honeydew, watermelon), nectarine, olive orange, clementine, mandarin, tangerine, papaya, peach, pear, persimmon, plantain, plum, prune (dried plum), pineapple, plumcot (or pluot), pomegranate, raspberry, salmonberry, star fruit, strawberry

Download free printable version at www.outsmartyourdiabetes.com/oyd-extras

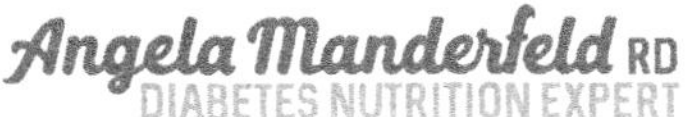

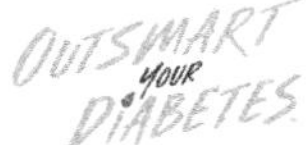

Now you have a new grocery list and guide to healing foods.

General Guidelines:

Aim for 5–9 servings of non starchy vegetables a day
Eat fish 2–3 times per week
Choose nuts, seeds, olive oil, and avocado as your healthy fats
Eat 2+ fruits a day
Aim for 25–40+g fiber a day
Gluten and dairy are optional depending on if there is a need to avoid, or not.

Supplements to consider:

Fish Oil, Turmeric, Ginger, CoQ10, Alpha Lipoic Acid, Vitamin D

Always talk to your provider before starting any supplements
as there could be interactions with medications.

References

Chapter 1

Marinac CR, Nelson SH, Breen CI, et al. Prolonged Nightly Fasting and Breast Cancer Prognosis. *JAMA Oncol*. 2016;2(8):1049-1055. doi:10.1001/jamaoncol.2016.0164

de Cabo R, Mattonson MP Effects of intermittent fasting on health, aging, and disease. *New England Journal of Medicine*, December 2019. https://www.nejm.org/doi/full/10.1056/NEJMra1905136

Chapter 2

De Fronzo, Ralph A. "From the Triumvirate to the Ominous Octet: A New Paradigm for the treatment of Type 2 Diabetes" Diabetes 2009 Apr: 58 (4): 773–795 "50% loss of beta cell function"

Diabetologia. "Diabetes may begin more than 20 years before diagnosis." ScienceDaily. Science Daily, 4 October 2018. <www.sciencedaily.com/releases/2018/10/181004192202.htm>

Saad MJ, Santos A, Prada PO. Linking Gut Microbiota and Inflammation to Obesity and Insulin Resistance.

Physiology (Bethesda). 2016;31(4):283-293. doi:10.1152/physiol.00041.2015

Chapter 3

American Diabetes Association. Economic Costs of Diabetes in the U.S. in 2017. Diabetes Care. 2018 May;41(5):917-928. DOI: 10.2337/dci18-0007.

Chapter 4

Rodríguez-Morán M, Guerrero-Romero F. Oral magnesium supplementation improves insulin sensitivity and metabolic control in type 2 diabetic subjects: a randomized double-blind controlled trial. Diabetes Care. 2003;26:1147−1152.

Amin MM, Asaad GF, Abdel Salam RM, El-Abhar HS, Arbid MS. Novel CoQ10 antidiabetic mechanisms underlie its positive effect: modulation of insulin and adiponectin receptors, Tyrosine kinase, PI3K, glucose transporters, sRAGE and visfatin in insulin resistant/diabetic rats. *PLoS One*. 2014;9(2):e89169. Published 2014 Feb 20. doi:10.1371/journal.pone.0089169

Zahedi H, Eghtesadi S, Seifirad S, et al. Effects of CoQ10 Supplementation on Lipid Profiles and Glycemic Control in Patients with Type 2 Diabetes: a randomized, double blind, placebo-controlled trial. *J Diabetes Metab Disord.* 2014;13:81. Published 2014 Jul 25. doi:10.1186/s40200-014-0081-6

Takikawa M, Inoue S, Horio F, Tsuda T. Dietary anthocyanin-rich bilberry extract ameliorates hyperglycemia and insulin sensitivity via activation of AMP-activated protein kinase in diabetic mice. *J Nutr.* 2010;140(3):527-533. doi:10.3945/jn.109.118216

Chapter 5

James J.DiNicolantonio, Sean C.Lucan, James H. O'Keefe "The Evidence for Saturated Fat and for Sugar Related to Coronary Heart Disease" Progress in Cardiovascular Diseases Volume 58, Issue 5, March–April 2016, Pages 464-472

Tatiana F.S. Teixeira, Maria Carmen Collado, Célia L.L.F. Ferreira, Josefina Bressan, Maria do Carmo G. Peluzio, "Potential mechanisms for the emerging link between obesity and increased intestinal permeability"Nutrition Research, Volume 32, Issue 9, 2012,Pages 637-647,ISSN 0271-5317, https://doi.org/10.1016/j.nutres.2012.07.003.

Khanum, A., Khan, S., Kausar, Samina, Mukhtar, F., Kausar Saima. Effects of Diaphragmatic Breathing Exercises on Blood Sugar Levels in Working Class Females with

Type-2 Diabetes Mellitus, Samina Kausar, Farhan Mukhtar and Saima Kausar, International Journal of Medical Research & Health Sciences, 2019, 8(1): 34-42 https://www.ijmrhs.com/medical-research/effects-of-diaphragmatic-breathing-exercises-on-blood-sugar-levels-in-working-class-females-with-type2-diabetes-mellitus.pdf

Mathiesen DS, Bagger JI, Bergmann NC, et al. The Effects of Dual GLP-1/GIP Receptor Agonism on Glucagon Secretion-A Review. *Int J Mol Sci*. 2019;20(17):4092. Published 2019 Aug 22. doi:10.3390/ijms20174092

Puhl RM, Heuer CA. Obesity stigma: important considerations for public health. *Am J Public Health*. 2010;100(6):1019-1028. doi:10.2105/AJPH.2009.159491

Monda V, Villano I, Messina A, et al. Exercise Modifies the Gut Microbiota with Positive Health Effects. *Oxid Med Cell Longev*. 2017;2017:3831972. doi:10.1155/2017/3831972 https://www.ncbi.nlm.nih.gov/pmc/articles/PMC5357536/

Daley CA, Abbott A, Doyle PS, Nader GA, Larson S. A review of fatty acid profiles and antioxidant content in grass-fed and grain-fed beef. *Nutr J*. 2010;9:10. Published 2010 Mar 10. doi:10.1186/1475-2891-9-10 https://www.ncbi.nlm.nih.gov/pmc/articles/PMC2846864/

Heart Outcomes Prevention Evaluation Study Investigators, Yusuf S, Dagenais G, Pogue J, Bosch J, Sleight P. Vitamin E supplementation and cardiovascular events in high-risk patients. N Engl J Med. 2000;342(3):154-160. doi:10.1056/NEJM200001203420302

Beulens JW, van der A DL, Grobbee DE, Sluijs I, Spijkerman AM, van der Schouw YT. Dietary phylloquinone and menaquinones intakes and risk of type 2 diabetes. *Diabetes Care*. 2010;33(8):1699-1705. doi:10.2337/dc09-2302

Bale BF, Doneen AL, Vigerust DJ. Precision Healthcare of Type 2 Diabetic Patients Through Implementation of Haptoglobin Genotyping. *Front Cardiovasc Med*. 2018;5:141. Published 2018 Oct 16. doi:10.3389/fcvm.2018.00141

Sofi F, Dinu M, Pagliai G, et al. Low-Calorie Vegetarian Versus Mediterranean Diets for Reducing Body Weight and Improving Cardiovascular Risk Profile: CARDIVEG Study (Cardiovascular Prevention With Vegetarian Diet). *Circulation*. 2018;137(11):1103-1113. doi:10.1161/CIRCULATIONAHA.117.030088

H. Dambha-Miller A. J. Day J. Strelitz G. Irving S. J. Griffin. Behaviour change, weight loss and remission of Type 2 diabetes: a community-based prospective cohort study. Diabet. Med. 37, 681– 688 (2020).

Lean ME, Leslie WS, Barnes AC, Brosnahan N, Thom G, McCombie L et al. Primary care-led weight management for remission of type 2 diabetes (DiRECT): an open-label, cluster-randomised trial. Lancet 2018; 391: 541– 551.

Lemieux I. Reversing Type 2 Diabetes: The Time for Lifestyle Medicine Has Come! Nutrients. 2020; 12(7):1974. https://doi.org/10.3390/nu12071974

Topping DL, Clifton PM. Short-chain fatty acids and human colonic function: roles of resistant starch and nonstarch polysaccharides. *Physiol Rev.* 2001;81(3):1031-1064. doi:10.1152/physrev.2001.81.3.1031

Alessandra Puddu, Roberta Sanguineti, Fabrizio Montecucco, Giorgio Luciano Viviani, "Evidence for the Gut Microbiota Short-Chain Fatty Acids as Key Pathophysiological Molecules Improving Diabetes", *Mediators of Inflammation*, vol. 2014, Article ID 162021, 9 pages, 2014. https://doi.org/10.1155/2014/162021

Bays H, Frestedt JL, Bell M, et al. Reduced viscosity Barley β-Glucan versus placebo: a randomized controlled trial of the effects on insulin sensitivity for individuals at risk for diabetes mellitus. *Nutr Metab (Lond)*. 2011;8:58. Published 2011 Aug 16. doi:10.1186/1743-7075-8-58

Chapter 6

Bradley Leech, Janet Schloss, Amie Steel, Association between increased intestinal permeability and disease: A systematic review. Advances in Integrative Medicine,Volume 6, Issue 1,2019,Pages 23-34, ISSN 2212-9588, https://doi.org/10.1016/j.aimed.2018.08.003.

Tanveer M, Ahmed A. Non-Celiac Gluten Sensitivity: A Systematic Review. *J Coll Physicians Surg Pak*. 2019;29(1):51-57. doi:10.29271/jcpsp.2019.01.51

Ohlsson B, Orho-Melander M, Nilsson PM. Higher Levels of Serum Zonulin May Rather Be Associated with Increased Risk of Obesity and Hyperlipidemia, Than with Gastrointestinal Symptoms or Disease Manifestations. *Int J Mol Sci*. 2017;18(3):582. Published 2017 Mar 8. doi:10.3390/ijms18030582

Fasano A. Zonulin and its regulation of intestinal barrier function: the biological door to inflammation, autoimmunity, and cancer. *Physiol Rev*. 2011;91(1):151-175. doi:10.1152/physrev.00003.2008

Fasano A, Berti I, Gerarduzzi T, et al. Prevalence of Celiac Disease in At-Risk and Not-At-Risk Groups in the United States: A Large Multicenter Study. Arch Intern Med. 2003;163(3):286–292. doi:10.1001/archinte.163.3.286

Bischoff SC, Barbara G, Buurman W, et al. Intestinal permeability--a new target for disease prevention and therapy. *BMC Gastroenterol*. 2014;14:189. Published 2014 Nov 18. doi:10.1186/s12876-014-0189-7

Tilg H, Moschen AR. Microbiota and diabetes: an evolving relationship. *Gut*. 2014;63(9):1513-1521. doi:10.1136/gutjnl-2014-306928

Müller, M., Hernández, M.A.G., Goossens, G.H. et al. Circulating but not faecal short-chain fatty acids are related to insulin sensitivity, lipolysis and GLP-1 concentrations in humans. Sci Rep 9, 12515 (2019). https://doi.org/10.1038/s41598-019-48775-0

Miller CK, Kristeller JL, Headings A, Nagaraja H, Miser WF. Comparative effectiveness of a mindful eating intervention to a diabetes self-management intervention among adults with type 2 diabetes: a pilot study. J Acad Nutr Diet. 2012;112(11):1835-1842. doi:10.1016/j.jand.2012.07.036

Gurung M, Li Z, You H, et al. Role of gut microbiota in type 2 diabetes pathophysiology. *EBioMedicine*. 2020;51:102590. doi:10.1016/j.ebiom.2019.11.051

Avena NM, Rada P, Hoebel BG. Evidence for sugar addiction: behavioral and neurochemical effects of intermittent, excessive sugar intake. *Neurosci Biobehav Rev*. 2008;32(1):20-39. doi:10.1016/j.neubiorev.2007.04.019

Sharma A, Amarnath S, Thulasimani M, Ramaswamy S. Artificial sweeteners as a sugar substitute: Are they really safe? Indian J Pharmacol. 2016 May-Jun;48(3):237-40. doi: 10.4103/0253-7613.182888. PMID: 27298490; PMCID: PMC4899993

Fowler SP, Williams K, Resendez RG, Hunt KJ, Hazuda HP, Stern MP. Fueling the obesity epidemic? Artificially sweetened beverage use and long-term weight gain. *Obesity (Silver Spring)*. 2008;16(8):1894-1900. doi:10.1038/oby.2008.284

Suez, J., Korem, T., Zeevi, D. *et al.* Artificial sweeteners induce glucose intolerance by altering the gut microbiota. *Nature* 514, 181–186 (2014). https://doi.org/10.1038/nature13793

Chapter 8

Eisele HJ, Markart P, Schulz R. Obstructive Sleep Apnea, Oxidative Stress, and Cardiovascular Disease: Evidence from Human Studies. *Oxid Med Cell Longev*. 2015;2015:608438. doi:10.1155/2015/608438Grace-FarfagliaP. Gluten and the Gut-Microbiota-Brain Axis: A Disturbance in the Force. EC Nutrition. 2015:236-238.

Bale BF, Doneen AL, Vigerust DJ. Precision Healthcare of Type 2 Diabetic Patients Through Implementation of Haptoglobin Genotyping. *Front Cardiovasc Med*. 2018;5:141. Published 2018 Oct 16. doi:10.3389/fcvm.2018.00141

Al Khatib HK, Harding SV, Darzi J, Pot GK. The effects of partial sleep deprivation on energy balance: a systematic review and meta-analysis. *Eur J Clin Nutr*. 2017;71(5):614-624. doi:10.1038/ejcn.2016.201

Li Y, Hao Y, Fan F, Zhang B. The Role of Microbiome in Insomnia, Circadian Disturbance and Depression. *Front Psychiatry*. 2018;9:669. Published 2018 Dec 5. doi:10.3389/fpsyt.2018.00669

Chapter 9

Ekelund U, Tarp J, Fagerland MW, et al Joint associations of accelero-meter measured physical activity and sedentary time with all-cause mortality: a harmonised meta-analysis in more than 44 000 middle-aged and older individuals. British Journal of Sports Medicine 2020;54:1499-1506.

Acknowledgments

To My Readers

I am inspired by you. You are what drives me to constantly learn and become a better practitioner. I truly appreciate the opportunities you have given me to be a part of your journey.

To My Family

Brad and Sam, I would not be where I am today if not for both of you. I am living my dream life as a wife, mother, and business owner. Not a day goes by that I don't recognize that my dreams have come true. Brad, thank you for helping me find balance in my many endeavors, for recognizing when and how I need to slow down, for providing your thoughtful wordsmithing talents in editing my book and, most of all, for supporting me in everything I do. It was your written word that brought us together and I thank you sincerely for editing mine.

To my mom, Beth, I am inspired and live in awe of the strength and determination with which you approach everything you do but particularly in reversing diabetes. You have been my biggest fan so, finally, here is the book you always said I would write.

To my dad, Rick, who taught me how to persevere and find the meaning of success.

To my sister, Kim, - my best friend who is always a source of laughter and fun.

To my Uncle Greg and grandparents, who trust and confide in me and allow me to support them in their diabetes journey as well. I am grateful for all of you.

To Camille, the best mother-in-law a woman could ask for. I owe you for a lifetime. Thank you for partnering with me on this wonderful and crazy adventure. Your careful crafting of sentences, your attention to detail and the countless hours you spent helping me edit this book are invaluable.

I love and thank you all!

To My Friends

To Jen, my awesome friend and accountability partner - thanks for always being an inspiration and helping me sort things out.

To Chere, my business coach and the things we've "attracted" together - you are amazing and I cannot thank you enough for helping me get to this point.

To all my diabetes colleagues to this point: Amy, Mindy, Julia,

Mary Lee, Bobbi, Judy, Ann Marie, Kena, Teresa, Angela, Meera, Luz, Maydelis. This list goes on and on but you all have been so important in getting me to where I am today.

To all my Zumba friends, you keep me going and grounded. You are my stress-relieving partners. Ana and Yongee, thanks for slowing me down on my "gerbil wheel." I'm grateful for you.

To My Publishing Team

To Stephanie, Jaci, Terri, Alyssa and Jerome, for creating such a beautiful cover, your skillful and thoughtful formatting, and your extensive knowledge on steps to self publishing were essential in helping my dream come to fruition.

To Colleen, for your editing and dietitian skills combined which gave me confidence that I was on the right track.

To Joshua, even though we have never met, you challenging me to write this in 30 days was really the only way this got done, very grateful for our paths crossing.

Many thanks to all!

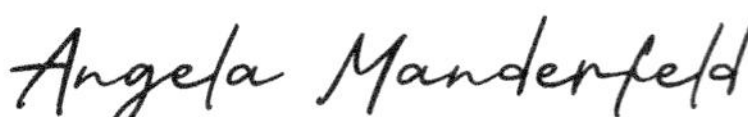

Angela Manderfeld RD

About the Author:

Angela Manderfeld is Registered Dietitian, Certified Diabetes Care and Education Specialist and Board Certified - Advanced Diabetes Management. Angela is a speaker, author, and clinician in private practice. She was introduced to integrative functional nutrition about eight years ago and has created programs to help her patients individualize their diabetes treatment to achieve lower blood sugar and more energy. Angela specializes in type 1 and type 2 diabetes with a special interest in continuous glucose monitors and insulin pumps. Her goal is to help her patients use food as medicine to improve their lives.

Working With Me

For more almost two decades I've been helping people like you outsmart diabetes.

This is not your typical diabetes program. We will get to the root cause of what is going on, you will receive highly individualized care, and education. It's time to stop focusing on dieting and start restoring your body to its original healthy state. No more fads, counting calories and measuring every bite. Learn to eat mindfully and integrate food as part of your healing process.

Your blood sugar will come down. You'll feel better, have more energy — and you'll need less medication.

Taking on diabetes or pre-diabetes can feel like enough of a challenge...

For your convenience, I deliver my services virtually. If you can sit in front of a computer when it's time for your appointment, you can work with me!

My Outsmart Your Diabetes Getting Started Program takes an integrative and functional nutrition approach to preventing, reversing, slowing or managing the progression of diabetes. Once we have looked closely at your lifestyle, discussed your goals and laid the groundwork, we will set the course for success.

Need a jumpstart for putting into practice what you have learned? Well, you can outsmart diabetes pretty easily, but you have to work a little harder to overcome your own habits. And, even when you do, it's not uncommon to get derailed. Things happen. Life gets stressful. Old patterns come back.

That's why I've broken it down into a simple two-week challenge. Change one habit a day for 14 days and, before you know it, your blood sugar will come down. Keep up those habits and — amazingly — it will stay down.

To be clear, diabetes is a chronic condition, so I'm not promising it's going to disappear altogether or that you can ditch your medication in a matter of weeks.

What I am saying is that you — yes you — can learn and maintain **14 key lifestyle habits that will help you get a handle on your diabetes once and for all.** If you take up the challenge and follow it consistently, you can expect even stubbornly high blood sugar levels to come back down.

You can do this 14 day challenge for FREE by signing up at www.outsmartyourdiabetes.com/oyd-extras/. It's my thank you for purchasing this book.

See programs and services at:
www.outsmartyourdiabetes.com

WORK WITH ME

Extra Credit for my A+ Readers

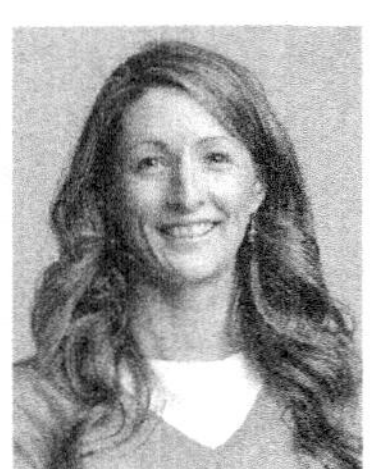

It's the back of the book!

You've come too far to be an armchair Outsmarter. Take what you've learned off the page and into real life.

Visit **www.outsmartyourdiabetes.com/oyd-extras** for bonuses and challenges to help you take the next step.

You'll Get:

- ✓ Printable copies of my worksheets you can use and reuse.
- ✓ Free admission to my guided 14 Day Blood Sugar Reboot, where you'll put everything you've learned into play.

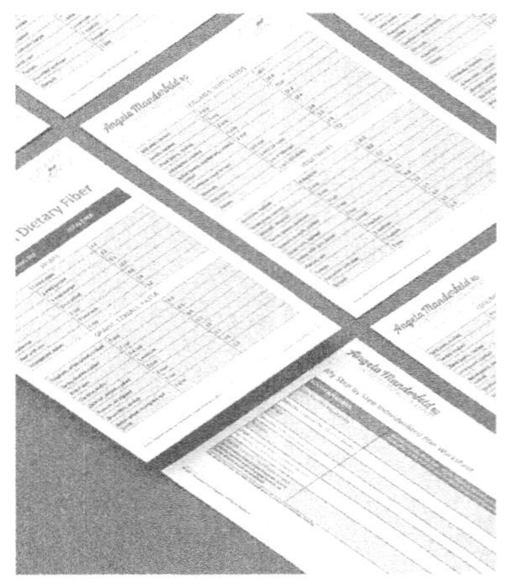

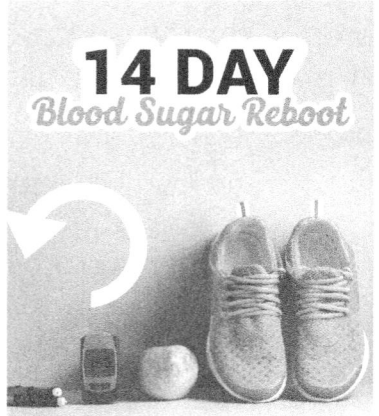

Index

A

B

C

D

E

F

G

H

I

J

K

L

M

N

O

P

Q

R

S

T

V

W

Y

Z